Prenatal

Parenting

To Vicki
In appreciation of all
you do for women with
less

[signature]

Prenatal Parenting

The Complete Psychological and Spiritual Guide to Loving Your Unborn Child

Frederick Wirth, M.D.

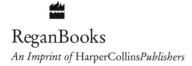

ReganBooks

An Imprint of HarperCollins*Publishers*

HarperCollins books may be purchased for educational, business, or sales promotional use. For information please write: Special Markets Department, HarperCollins Publishers Inc., 10 East 53rd Street, New York, NY 10022.

FIRST EDITION

Designed by Nancy Singer Olaguera

Printed on acid-free paper

Library of Congress Cataloging-in-Publication Data

Wirth, Frederick.
    Prenatal parenting / Frederick Wirth.—1st ed.
        p.   cm.
    Includes bibliographical references and index.
    ISBN 0-06-039422-6
        1. Prenatal care—Handbooks, manuals, etc. 2. Fetus—Growth—
    Handbooks, manuals, etc. 3. Pregnancy—Handbooks, manuals,
    etc. I. Title.
RG940 .W56 2001
618.2'4—dc21
                                                        2001019403

01 02 03 04 05 ❖/RRD 10 9 8 7 6 5 4 3 2 1

To my parents, who gave me unconditional love,
and to my children and patients, who taught me
about the work of love

Contents

Acknowledgments

The thoughts in this book come from the wisdom of many dedicated people who make the effort to teach. I have benefited by learning from them all. My life is enriched by my learning the wisdom of living with abundant love from my wife, Linda, who is my steadfast beacon of hope and joy through life's dark valleys.

I am also grateful for the wordsmith skills of my editors, Doug Corcoran and Allison St. Claire; and for my agent, Margret McBride, and her able associate, Kris Wallace, who enthusiastically introduced this book to the daunting world of publishing.

The love and support of steadfast friends gave me the energy to persevere and write this book while facing many distractions. These included Lois and Lenny Lax, Dr. Walter Cohen, Pat and Peter Binnion, Art and Pat Baer, Maureen and Frank McGrath, Kent Lawrence, Bill and Keith Dozier, Fred and Irene Shabel, Kay Templeton, Jackie Osmond, William and Anne Hoskins, George and Melissa Vosburgh, Captain Kathy Hobbs, Ricki Baker, and Jeanette Finkle. They all enthusiastically gave their loyal support to this project.

$\mathcal{P}$reface

We love because it is the only true adventure.

—Nikki Giovanni

For twenty-six years I have been rescuing premature infants, spending six- and twelve-hour vigils by their bedsides, giving my all and all that modern medical science has to offer my tiny patients. I know that I am working with the world's greatest medical resources, and yet I am frustrated. I have the knowledge, the skills, the medications, and the medical technology to offer my two-pound patients the best chance of surviving their life-threatening predicaments, but it is so disheartening to know that some of these awful starts in life were preventable.

All of us around my patient's bed—parents, nurses, technicians, and colleagues—know that this fragile new child is an innocent victim struggling against life-threatening events that have brought him pain and suffering maybe for the rest of his life. I watch helplessly as he depletes his metabolic stores while working with all his strength to inhale his next breath. Although his breathing is assisted by ventilators, muscle stimulants, and IV nutrition, being born too early presents too many obstacles to overcome. He slowly loses his strength, periodically stopping his breathing, too fatigued from the work of staying alive. A gentle tap on his foot or a soft stroke to his back stimulates him to take a few more breaths.

Inevitably, more and more stimulus is needed, as the periods of not breathing become more frequent. The tone of his tiny muscles evaporates. His energy sapped, this tiny baby is now limp, nearly lifeless, a perfectly formed infant slowly and painfully losing his struggle against premature birth.

My work of caring for critically ill premature infants became so painful that twenty years ago I pushed away from my myopic view of putting more and more effort and money into the rescue of prematurely born infants one by one and redirected my efforts toward helping more women carry their pregnancies to term. I searched the world's literature, talked with my respected colleagues, and came to the following conclusions.

The United States has the best and most expensive medical system, but my medical specialty of neonatal-perinatal medicine is not getting the job done. My obstetrical colleagues are expertly trained, have the best equipment, and are doing world-class research, but there are some distressing national statistics that embarrass me professionally.

The mortality rate for American babies under one year of age is higher than that of any other Western industrialized nation in the world.[1] This horrible statistic exists in spite of the fact that we spend more money per person on health care than any other nation. What is interesting (if you can say that about this disturbing topic) is that once an infant is delivered prematurely, and is cared for in an intensive care nursery, the chances of her survival are as good in the United States as in any other nation.[2]

The questions then arise: Why are we ranked so poorly in the world in infant mortality, and why has the rate of premature births continued to increase for the past twenty-five years in this country, while it has decreased in other industrially developed nations?

The answer is simple. The science of obstetrics is not designed or structured to reduce the incidence of premature births. Your prenatal visits and most of the lab work that goes along with them primarily help your health care provider recognize complications of pregnancy that might threaten your health and/or the health of your unborn infant.

The solution to reducing the number of babies born before term, however, is not simple. The great thinkers in the obstetrical departments of the finest universities in this country are working hard to find a medical cure for preterm births. But we still have not made much progress in solving the problem medically.

I have watched as one infant after another was admitted to the intensive care units I have directed. Each time I wondered, What went wrong? Why is this infant here? Can all this pain, suffering, and expense be avoided? After hours of work stabilizing each of my tiny, frail patients, I returned to their mothers' charts and talked with their concerned obstetricians and families. Typically, I found health problems or the presence of risky behavior that should been attended to or controlled. If only the mothers knew more. If only they and their families had the necessary knowledge and skills, these tragic events could have been prevented.

Every baby deserves a good birth, one that allows her to develop to her genetic potential. Tears well up in my eyes and my heart becomes heavy whenever my wife, Linda, and I see a child struggling with the life-long handicaps from a premature birth. Linda will feel my unspoken anguish and ask what is wrong. All I can do is nod my head in the direction of the wheelchair-bound child, tended by a loving family. Nothing more needs to be said between us. We both know the magnitude of the daily sacrifices made by these families—sacrifices those of us more fortunate have never had to make because our children were born healthy. She knows that I can neither watch nor approach this family for fear of becoming too emotional in front of them and upsetting their family outing. Times like this bring my thoughts back to the countless chart reviews that have clearly shown me how such tragedies can be prevented.

Many patients believe that the outcome of their pregnancy depends solely on the quality of their medical care. This is not true. The quality of your pregnancy outcome also depends on the psychological and spiritual content of your life. Only you and your family are capable of managing many of the various risks that can adversely affect the outcome of your pregnancy. Risky behaviors such as using alcohol, tobacco, or illicit drugs are commonly discussed during prenatal care, but they represent only a few of the risks to your unborn child. There are many more risks, such as not expressing your emotions, negative self-talk, low self-esteem, not talking to your unborn child, and not knowing how to be your best under stress. This book is about how to make psychological and spiritual changes that will help you exercise and work safely, manage pain and fear successfully, and effectively parent your unborn child. This is what sets this book apart from others.

This book is dedicated to preparing you for the great life adventure of birthing a baby, a quest of great proportions that will transform you and your family. You, the champion of this quest—just like the prototypical literary hero—must overcome many new challenges during the pregnancy and childrearing that follows.

Classic quest stories are told in all of the world's cultures to impart important messages to their people. Each venture begins with an unexpected call, a yearning for something more, which stirs a person into action. This begins a journey filled with new and often challenging experiences that confront the hero or heroine with one calamity after another. But the traveler prevails, overcoming all obstacles to proceed toward the quest's goal.

Throughout the adventure, the traveler makes the commitment to endure whatever is necessary to obtain the goal of a rich treasure, for example. But at the same time, the quest always transforms the hero or heroine into someone better who has gained the real treasure: new knowledge or an expanded, life-changing awareness that is far more valuable than the physical goal of the quest.

We all grow up hearing these popular stories that transcend time and culture. They strike an important chord of recognition because we all face challenges in our lives. The world's great storytellers use the outside, physical world to relate truths about our internal world—our fears, our beliefs, and our triumphs over life obstacles—all of which make up our character, our ability to withstand hardship, to work and make sacrifices for a higher ideal.

During your pregnancy you will face fears about the welfare of your developing fetus, pain during labor, and possibly your ability to care properly for your baby after her birth. Your beliefs, how you think and feel about your world, and how you judge your ability to handle these challenges are very important to your pregnancy's success. This book will guide you through the development of important concepts about faith and self-esteem, as well as the scientific information about the benefits of meditation and prayer.

Birthing a baby is obviously a quest of epic proportions for a family. You will face transformational challenges that will call upon all of your internal resources and powers. Your external prize will be a wondrous baby, and your internal treasure will be a new commitment to protecting and nourishing this new miracle.

You and your family are the heroes in the pregnancy quest. I am the trailblazer, a companion who is a helper, for your adventure. I will show the way during difficult times. I will be there when you have questions and need help in achieving your goal of a safe pregnancy and a healthy baby. But the real work of overcoming the challenges of the pregnancy is up to you and your family. As a trailblazer, I have my own quest as we go along this adventure together. My goal is to empower you with information so you will understand what is going on with your body, your mind, your fetus, your partner, your family, and, finally, with your health care provider and delivery facility. I will help you conclude this pregnancy with excitement, joy, and the great expectation of achieving your goal in this incredible adventure.

There is no better gift you can give your child than a safe pregnancy. It is the gift of life that lasts a lifetime. What a blessing for your child. What a privilege for you!

This book is my message to couples about how to prevent a family tragedy of inestimable proportions from happening to them. I dedicate this work to my patients and their loving families who struggle daily against the legacies of being born too early. I have learned much from them.

For the past twenty-five years I have been a trailblazer for many birthing families, and they tell me wonderful tales of their triumphs over adversities, whether it was overcoming the fear of childbirth pain, stopping risky behaviors, developing new relationships with their family members, or their newfound capacity to nurture and love. There is a better way! You will be amazed, as I and thousands of my patients have been, at the wonderful difference it makes after the infant's birth.

Yes, you can make a difference. By reading and practicing the simple exercises presented, you will gain the self-confidence and the know-how to greatly enhance your own health, and that of your unborn baby.

Let's begin that beautiful journey.

Part I

Fetal Parenting

1

$\mathcal{T}$ake a Fetal Love Break

A man's mother is his other God.

—*African proverb*

The phone rings and I awake from a deep sleep. An anxious voice says that I am needed in Room 129 for a Baby Boy W in fetal distress. Immediately my heart rate accelerates as I shake the sleep from my not-yet-fully-alert mind. As I walk down the short hall to the delivery room, I prepare mentally to be at my best for this innocent infant going through a major life crisis that will test his physiologic reserves.

When I arrive, I get a quick report from his mother's doctor. His eyes are tired and his voice tense as he tells me that he must deliver this infant as soon as possible and it's too late to try for a C-section. I glance at the fetal heart monitor, and see the all-too-familiar heart rate pattern of a fetus in distress.

After checking with the nurses on my resuscitation team to be sure everything we need is present and in order, I notice for the first time the embrace between my little patient's mother and her life partner. They are face-to-face with the father's arms around her shoulders. He is whispering in her ear while she recovers from the last uterine contraction.

Her obstetrician interrupts them to give the urgent message that he needs her full cooperation and a maximal effort to push her infant out during the next contraction. The contraction comes and with deep concentration and intention, she bears down with all her might. She is obviously reaching deep within herself to deliver her baby's head now, before it is too late.

Her husband has risen from his embrace to count the interval between her breaths. They are working as a team that has obviously practiced this cadence many times. Together they are successful in pushing out the infant's head.

Her doctor quickly notices the umbilical cord is tightly wrapped around the baby's neck. He deftly clamps and cuts the cord, which interrupts the only oxygen available to the infant. Now there is no chance for the infant to recover until after the delivery, when ventilation is established.

It's my responsibility to assist the infant in making this important transition to good ventilation with plenty of oxygen. It is now a race against the accelerating biological damage that occurs when his vital organs don't have enough oxygen.

Once the chest is delivered, I notice his slate-gray skin color—one of the cardinal signs of asphyxia, a condition that can cause permanent brain damage. I feel the effects of an adrenaline surge in my own body. Everyone in the room is tense. We all have the same wishful mind-set. Please dear baby, take a breath.

Like an answered prayer, he takes his first breath, and then begins to cry as the obstetrician dries him off with a sterile towel. I quickly suction his mouth and nose and do a cursory assessment of his clinical condition. Once I am sure he no longer needs additional oxygen and his cardiovascular system is stable, I swaddle him and carry him to the open arms of his parents.

Up to this moment his facial expression was a contorted grimace. He had experienced profound physiologic stress, and the survival of many vital organs systems was at risk. Once he hears the words of endearment from his parents, his facial expression changes. He relaxes his grimace. There is a slight change in the tilt of his head and I notice the drop in the hunch of his shoulders.

A few minutes later he opens his eyes and looks directly at his mother's face. Again his expression changes and there is a wide intense gaze of excitement, which captures his parents' ardent attention as they stroke and talk to him. Slowly and barely perceptibly his face melts into an angelic smile of contentment.

An expression of such endearment always creates an emotional release in me. I am assured that once again the miraculous biology of the newborn infant has withstood the vagaries of hypoxia and asphyxia that certainly would have killed any adult. Yet in minutes, he is at peace and in obvious full recovery.

No one fully understands why the newborn can recover so quickly and completely from these severe physiologic insults, but each of us in neonatal medicine appreciates and respects the biology of the human reproductive system. We revere the capacity of the newborn to withstand immense biological stress. Each time I observe their recovery capacity, I thank God for allowing me once again to witness this miracle.

Most movies and novels depict the discovery of pregnancy as a wonderful, joyous event that miraculously changes the couple's lives and their relationship. This romantic view of pregnancy may or may not be true for you. Many couples are surprised by the news that they are pregnant. Some are prepared, some are not, and some may be upset by an unplanned pregnancy.

Pregnancy is a time of change and challenge. It is a time when we reevaluate our attitudes and priorities. It is a time of great personal growth and interesting opportunities.

I was surprised and perplexed by the announcement that we were pregnant with all four of our children. I was not overwhelmed but indeed amazed that the pregnancy had occurred. My life did not change overnight. My wife and I did not find new joy at the discovery of the pregnancy. Instead of celebrating, I started thinking about the new responsibilities—both personally and financially. I also was frightened by all the possible complications of pregnancy, and the dangers that both my wife and unborn child faced. After all, I deal with those complications twenty-four hours a day in my work. It wasn't until my first birth that I really got into the magic of being a parent.

I now realize that I missed a great opportunity both for me and my children. I should have switched from being the worried provider to being the nurturer for my wife and developing child. Like most people, I didn't know about the amazing capacity of my children to receive love while developing in their mother's womb. There are so many ways we parents can love and nurture our unborn children. This book will guide you through this important parenting role and offer valuable exercises to give your unborn child the magical gift of love—a gift, you will learn, that has the potential to change your child's life in incredible ways.

Let's first look at ten little-known facts about a fetus.[1]

1. A fetus has more nerve cells and many more connections among them than an adult.
2. He has a memory of his experiences before birth.
3. He develops consciousness and a sense of self separate from his mother before birth.
4. He can hear, smell, taste, and see before birth.
5. His in utero experience builds the brain architecture that will determine his behavior after birth and probably for the rest of his life.
6. He communicates with his mother biochemically as well as through his senses.
7. He shares his mother's emotional experiences.
8. His mother cannot hide her most intimate thoughts and feelings from him.
9. He is born looking for meaningful relationships and knows how to develop them.
10. Each infant is born with a distinct temperament that may require specific parenting techniques for proper nurturing after birth.

Everything you think, feel, and do while pregnant has a profound impact on your child both before and after birth. You are a brain shaper, a life shaper. Your role as a loving, powerful parent begins long before your baby's first cry or smile.

By the time the fetus has completed the twelfth week of gestation, the total number of neurons he will have for the rest of his life have already formed. By the time he is twenty-eight weeks old, he has developed all of his senses as well as those brain parts dedicated to emotional responses and memory. By this time in gestation, the unborn infant is developing concepts about himself and the world in which his mother lives.

And what about that newborn child? Consider this.

The newborn infant is the most intelligent organism in the universe. His brain has greater flexibility and a larger learning capacity than an adult's brain. Immediately after birth, he is constantly exploring his new environment and experimenting with new ways to interact effectively with all that he experiences. He continually tries new behaviors and closely watches the reactions of the people around him. He changes his behaviors and compares the new reactions to the old ones and modifies his experiments by a continuing feedback loop of information that he evaluates and remembers. By using these developed techniques he gets what he deems is important, which in most cases is the attention of his parents.[2]

This exploration actually starts twelve weeks prior to birth and continues until the child reaches his second birthday. After this critical period of brain development, the learning capabilities and flexibility of the child's brain diminish. These experiences during these important twenty-seven months actually shape the architecture and biochemistry of his developing brain.

The child who experiences love and security will respond to new situations with confidence and wonder, while the child who experiences abuse and neglect will respond to the same situation with anxiety and vigilance. At conception, if there is no use of illicit drugs, alcohol, or tobacco, the brains of these two children had the same potential. By their second birthday, the architecture and biochemistry of these two brains are completely different. One child's brain is wired to explore and learn, while the other's is organized to be leery of pain and neglect.[3]

The child who experiences security and love develops a brain with a biochemistry and architecture that welcomes new information. He is highly curious and constantly explores his enchanted environment. His early experiences set him on the road to developing confidence, high self-esteem, and a relaxed approach to new situations, which greatly enhance his ability to learn.

The early responses in the neglected child's brain tend to repeat themselves and are reinforced until the child is conditioned to be hyperalert to danger. All other information irrelevant to the perceived danger is filtered by his brain as unimportant. Over time these early responses grow into impulsive, violent ones that typically lead the young adolescent into criminal activity.

By choosing this book, I know which type of child you would prefer. Congratulations! Let's start a fascinating journey together to create your successful, healthy pregnancy and child.

Start with Yourself

You will need to think and write about what you read in these pages. So let a pen and notebook be your companions while reading this book. Your writings will begin as notes and become your pregnancy journal, as significant a keepsake as a baby book. It will be a record of the events, thoughts, and feelings you experience during this pregnancy, and it will become a record of your progress in building the skills needed to make yours a positive, safe pregnancy. Even better would be for both you and the baby's father to do the various written exercises, and then compare notes and share your thoughts with each other. You'll gain incredibly valuable insights and develop an excellent foundation for birthing and raising your unborn child. I call these interludes with your unborn child *fetal love breaks.*

A journaling technique I have found very powerful is called "sentence stemming," in which you complete a number of sentences with as many answers as flow into your mind. It's a remarkable way to explore your unconscious mind, which is a wellspring of intuitive knowledge for you and your developing child.[4]

At the top of a page in your journal, write each of the sentence stems I list for you, and then quickly write seven to ten endings to the sentences as they come to mind without any thought of censorship or logic. Write quickly. Don't worry about what you are writing, even when your endings may be contradictory. Worrying will block the process of getting on paper the genius of your mind. Once the idea or sentence is on paper, you can go back and evaluate it.

If you are unable to give a quick answer, or can complete only a few, put the pen and paper aside, relax, and then come back to the sentence stems later. This is an excellent way to explore your unconscious feelings about these topics.

When doing sentence stemming, I am amazed at the wisdom of my unconscious mind. What usually happens is that a few endings come to mind immediately, but the important ones come later, when I am reaching to think of another. It is important not to give up writing your sentence endings when you feel blocked. Just keep writing whatever comes to your mind, including "I have nothing else to write."

Now, explore your feelings around the time you first heard about being pregnant by completing these sentence stems.

When I first learned about my pregnancy, I felt . . .

When my life partner learned about the pregnancy, she/he felt . . .

A child in my life will . . . to my relationship with my life partner.

At this time a child in my life will . . .

The gifts I want to give my child . . .

What I can do now to nurture and love my child . . .

After completing this exercise, look over what you have written. See if any new thoughts come to mind. You will want to come back to this first exercise later in the book to review your progress in thinking. You will change. I did when my wife was pregnant. All families do. The word *pregnancy* means an abundant time rich with important possibilities for you, your family, and your unborn child. That is why it is important to do the love work presented in this book. We'll examine the enormously important aspects of pregnancy: physical, emotional, and spiritual. We'll look at the powerful role of negative feelings such as fear or self-doubt and how to turn negative behaviors into positive feelings and actions. You'll learn how to take control of your life in order to offer the best start in life to your baby.

It's an exciting, often challenging experience. And I know you can do it.

2

Communicating with Your Unborn Child

Before you were conceived I wanted you
Before you were born I loved you
Before you were here an hour I would die for you
This is the miracle of life.

—Maureen Hawkins

I am blessed with a job that makes a difference. Each morning I get out of bed knowing that the work I do will affect someone's life for perhaps seventy-five years. This is exciting and rewarding, but my job also comes with burdens. There is so much to learn and do—all of it important.

In spite of the glamour of my hospital setting, I am humbled by what I experience. At work, I feel like the pen in the hand of a great author writing meaningful words. The knowledge I possess was fed to me by many dedicated teachers. They organized and offered me the marvelous gift of wisdom collected over the centuries of mankind toiling with the sick and injured. The hand of this wisdom guides me as its instrument to create the miracles I watch daily. Once the work is done, I, like the great author's pen, am put down until needed again. I am no more or less important than that pen. How well I do my job affects my patient's future, but the healing benefits they receive pass through me like thoughts passing through an

10

author's pen. My reward comes from experiencing the miracle of the biology that heals my tiny, born-too-soon patients.

I now use a pen to write from my experience and hope that you will become conscious of the wonder of God's creation in you. You, too, can benefit from the collective wisdom of many dedicated researchers and health care providers. It is up to you to seize this opportunity with conviction, excitement, and optimism. This is your gift to your unborn child that no one else can give. My prayer is that the information you're about to read will either change or clarify the way you think and feel about yourself, your God, and the universe in which you live.

The first, and most important, significant finding for you to learn is that what you believe and how you think changes the connections between your nerve cells and the biochemistry of your mind and body.[1] "The word became flesh" as written in the Bible is literally true.[2] Neuroscientists have proved that words, music, emotions, and experience all change the wiring in our brains as well as the chemistry of our bodies. I am confronted daily by this fantastic fact as I observe the behavior of my patients.

We know that the shape and architecture of premature infants' brains are sculpted by what they experience in the intensive care nursery as well as in utero. This alteration in their brains' wiring affects how they react later in life. It determines their temperament and ability to do complex thinking.[3]

What is even more compelling is that my patients' brain building is driven by the quality of the relationships they have with their parents and with health care providers. My patients are so skillful in connecting with me and reading my nonverbal cues that they know how I feel and think about them. They constantly experiment with new behaviors and techniques to connect with me, and if I or, more important, their parents, fail to respond, they eventually run out of energy from trying too hard and shut down biochemically, at great cost to their emotional and intellectual development. The cognitive and emotional content of the nursery experience matters. The younger the patient, the more potent the experience is in determining the infant's developing personality and intellect.[4] We caregivers are baby brain builders, and so are you. What a daunting responsibility!

What I watch happening to my patients in the nursery is first happening to your baby in utero. I am caring for and loving infants born as early as twenty-three weeks after conception. I have witnessed the well-organized nervous system of a baby born after a twenty-three- to twenty-four-week gestation become disorganized by his experience in his new unnatural environment in my nursery. I have seen contented well-coordinated infants, who were at peace before delivery, become irritable, aggressive, hyperactive infants who grimace each time I approach. A baby who was once easily consoled by a gentle touch or by his mother's voice, within days after his birth may need medical sedation with drugs to calm him. Without the sedating medication, he fights the ventilator and the nurses caring for him until he runs out of energy and collapses into a listless state of fatigue.

This distresses me greatly, because I know this experience is setting the tone of how he will interact with his environment and people for the rest of his life. Studies have shown convincingly that these behaviors persist into the school-age years. Most of my patients survive their intensive care nursery experience with normal intelligence, but many will have problems with school performance because of poor interpersonal skills, impulsiveness, distractibility, and other neurological handicaps that interfere with concentrating on and completing assignments.[5]

I attend weeklong international conferences to learn how to observe and react to the needs of my tiny patients while they are in the intensive care nursery. I am learning to recognize which infants are in extreme stress and how to help them reorganize their brains. I want each and every parent also to know how to do this for their unborn and/or newborn child if needed. Research clearly shows that what we do in the early stages of their lives determines how well they will do in school and later in life.[6]

My tiny patients are seeking human contact. They know how to get it. All one has to do is look into their worried, inquisitive faces to see how intense this need is. I have learned to communicate with these infants by reading their facial and body cues. I had to attend professional seminars to learn this skill, but babies are born already knowing all about it. They watch us carefully for facial cues and sounds that reassure them they are loved. On my daily rounds I ask my nurses, "What is your patient saying to you today?" We can tell when they are content and relaxed, or when they are anxious and distressed. We know when they are in pain and when they are hungry. We can also discern the difference in them when their parents arrive in the nursery.

My patients respond to my voice, gentle touch, and love, but all my knowledge and skill are not as powerful as their parents' voice and touch. I have witnessed over and over the powerful healing effects of a mother's soothing touch and loving words. Parents know this instinctually and now medical science is finally catching on. Medical researchers have realized that a baby recognizes his mother's voice and smell, and these stimuli tell the brain to pay attention, this person is important.

What is happening in my intensive care nursery between parents and my patients is happening between you and your unborn child. She is responding to your voice and to your every thought and emotion. The connection between you and your unborn child is so powerful that it is impossible to hide your thoughts or feelings from her.

Your brain is much more than a collection of nerves genetically organized to operate your body. It also secretes numerous chemicals called neuropeptides. The composition of these neuropeptides in your bloodstream affects your emotions, your perceptions of what is happening in your environment, and how most of our organs function, such as our immune and digestive systems, over which we have no direct conscious control. These neuropeptides are messenger molecules. They control your thoughts, your emotions, and your memories. They helped determine your brain development. They affect how you reacted to all your experiences.[7] The vital point? These messenger molecules cross the placenta to bathe the developing brain and body of your unborn child. As they affect your reactions to life experiences, they help determine the brain development of your unborn child and will affect how he reacts to every experience he will face in life.

The deterioration of my tiny patient's brain after his premature birth is caused by his sensory experience in the busy, noisy, brightly lit intensive care nursery. He was a competent fetus minutes before I held him in my hands, but within hours I notice his behavior, muscle tone, and reflexes change because of the stress of being born too early. Then my colleagues and I watch as this brave, hearty little patient tries to recover. He can do it with lots of help from people who love and care for him. We don't know exactly how to prevent the deterioration in his behavior, but we believe every experience counts.

What is even more important is that you, dear reader, are the first and most powerful influence in shaping your baby's brain. You have much more power than I to be the architect of your developing baby's brain. What you think, feel, and say all change the synaptic connections in your baby's nervous system. This knowledge may be frightening because of its awesome responsibility, but I hope you'll see it as a magnificent opportunity for positive good.

The Wonder of It All

Science is waking to the idea that the infant's mind is an amazing organ. In fact, it is the universe's most amazing organ. There's an unfortunate misconception in our culture that infancy is a grace period of relative ease and a prelude to the important period of real brain development during the school years. Some mistakenly see babyhood as the developmental period for learning basic muscle control and all parents have to do is meet the infant's basic needs of nutrition and safety. For years the conventional wisdom about babies was that they had no emotions and were genetically set to mature on a predetermined schedule. Medical science was fixed on the paradigm of infants' minds as blank slates. Most parents knew better than that, but scientists ignored their observations that children had different temperaments at birth and recognized their parents' faces and voices.

Just the reverse is true. Infants' learning capabilities surpass our brightest college students. They think, observe, and reason. They consider evidence, do experiments to verify their hypotheses, draw conclusions from their observations, and search for truth. They know lots about their world and actively seek new information. They continually repeat this process of scientific investigation until they get the reaction they are seeking.

Babies predict a reaction for each action they take. If the expected does not happen, they quickly discard the nonvalid theory and develop a new one. This is the period of most rapid growth and development not only in muscle control, but also in emotional control that is the foundation of how they will relate to people in the future. Babies have been doing this scientific work for centuries, while scientists only developed their methods during the last five hundred years. Scientists are good learners when they use the same techniques babies use.[8]

Here are some of the amazing things newborns learn during the first few hours after birth. Within minutes of seeing his mother a newborn can pick out her face from a gallery of many faces. Infants can pick out the sex of other babies by the way they move even when dressed. Newborn infants can imitate facial expressions. They do not have to experiment with this. They just do it.

Babies coordinate their own expressions with others. Their voices and gestures mimic us. They literally flirt and have perfect timing. They want our attention and know how to get it. When you talk, your baby becomes still, and when you stop, his movements pick up with kicking legs and waving fists. Babies form close relationships with their caregivers. They express themselves, exhibit preferences, and influence people from the very beginning.

Within months they can recognize the emotions of their caregiver by reading body cues. They can match a recording of a sad voice with a picture of a sad face but will become confused and frustrated if the voice does not match the face.

So, What Role Do Our Genes Play?

I was taught in medical school that a child fortunate enough to be birthed by intelligent parents had a good chance of inheriting a high IQ as an adult. Back then, scientists thought brain development was set by genetic endowment that was not affected by outside stimulation. Today, research with new imaging capabilities has clearly shown the contrary. Brain development is far from being preset by genetic code. Human brain development is unlike the development of any other organ in our body. The architecture and function of the human brain are determined by a combination of genetic endowment and the environment in which it develops before and after birth.[9] Ninety-nine percent of our genetic material is identical to that of a chimpanzee, yet we act and develop differently from the chimpanzee.[10] One obvious example is that we are able to live in many different climates, while apes and monkeys live in restricted ecological niches. (And, unfortunately, many of them may become extinct because of their inability to adapt to other areas.) There is only one species of humans, and we successfully live in all the earth's ecological systems, including the bottom of the ocean and outer space for limited periods. Why have we been so successful when our next of kin from a genetic point of view is having so much trouble?

One obvious answer is that our brain outperforms the chimp's, but there is no way we can explain the differences between our intellect and success as a species by just a 1 percent difference in our genetic makeup. There is a great difference in the size and shape of our brains. The human brain's frontal lobe is much larger than the chimp's, and evolutionists think this is what makes us human. This is the area of the brain where we do our most critical thinking, such as deciding the appropriateness of behaviors.

We are able to do this not by our genetic makeup, but by our ability to engineer our own brain to help us adapt to our birth environment. Scientists tell us that roughly 60 percent of our genes are dedicated to our brain development. Our genetic code is important for the lower centers of the brain that maintain our body's physiologic functions such as respiration and pulse rates, but in the development of the cortex, genes direct the brain to produce as many cells and connections it can to set the brain's framework, and our environment and early experiences then shape the neurocircuits. The brain organizes itself around its experience. Everything the fetus or infant experiences affects his brain's architecture and function.

Developmental specialists have long understood that embryos are not simply small, unformed versions of adults, but they have not fully understood how well the embryo adapts to the intrauterine environment. Human embryos and fetuses have special physiologic capacities that help them adapt to the changing challenges of intrauterine life. Yet the behavioral sciences are just beginning to understand this concept as it relates to childhood neurodevelopment and adult behaviors.

The genetic material we inherit from our parents can be beneficially or adversely impacted by our fetal experience in the womb. The interplay between the fetal genetic makeup and the intrauterine environment gives the fetus a greater opportunity to survive adverse prenatal events; however, there is a lifelong price to pay if the fetus has to take protective action to adapt to adverse prenatal conditions. For example, babies who develop in an unfavorable prenatal condition of maternal malnutrition are more prone to heart disease, obesity, and altered stress responses in their life, although these effects may not appear until the stressed fetus reaches middle age.[11]

More Common Misconceptions About What Our Genes Do

Most people think that particular traits are caused solely by genetics. Like most doctors, I was trained to believe that my genes determined how I would perform in life. If we are fortunate to have parents with good genes and then lucky enough to take the positive draw of genes from one parent over the other, we are likely to have a more successful life.

I was thankful that I inherited my mother's temperament and my father's drive and work ethic. Actually, the only truth is that my hair color came from my mother. The other more important characteristics of my behavior and general health are a combination of my gene pool and what happened to me in utero and for the first two years after my birth. Now that I am aware of how important it was for my parents to nurture me in the way they did and how that love affected my productivity and success even at this stage in my life, I am enormously grateful for what they did for me.

Prenatal programming, which is the combination of our genetic endowment from our parents and our intrauterine environment, affects how we perform mentally and physically during life. The most fantastic and provocative discovery to come out of neuroscience laboratories is that the fetal and infant brain thrives on feedback from its environment. It wires itself into a thinking and emotional organ from what it experiences. This prenatal programming is why no two brains are exactly alike, including those of identical twins.[12]

The question of nature versus nurture is complex, but now the debate is over. Both play a major role in neurological and psychological development. The traits we have are a combination of our genetic makeup and our prenatal and postnatal environments. But, most important, the nurturer of a fetus or infant is a brain builder.

3

On Becoming a Brain Architect

Children must be taught how to think, not what to think.
—*Margaret Mead*

Fetal brain growth and development are so complex that little was written about them until the advent of advanced imaging techniques during this age of medical technology. A major misconception is that our brain is a complex system of wires that function similar to a giant supercomputer. Computers are completely wired before they are turned on. Our brain is so much more. It continually rewires itself long after it has started functioning. It also produces many neuropeptides that affect all our organs. Our brain is a living, dynamic organ that keeps adapting to its ever-changing environment.

The fetal brain develops in stages. This starts with its simpler, more primitive parts located in the brain's center and finishes with its extremely complex convoluted cortex. The first part to develop in utero is the brain stem, which regulates basic body functions such as heart rate and temperature. It sits atop the spinal cord and its final structure and function are determined primarily by our genes. The second stage to develop is called the midbrain, which controls sleep, appetite, and arousal. This is followed by the limbic system, which is the center for emotional control. Finally, the last to develop is the cortex, the seat of rational thinking and analytical process. As each more complex stage develops, the fetal environment and experience become more important in determining its structure and function. In fact, the limbic system and cortex continue to change structure and function long after birth.

During this progression of brain development, each developed part regulates the development of subsequent stages. For example, if a mother uses drugs while the brain stem or midbrain are developing, it will have major impact on the limbic system and cortex, which develop later.

The developmental stages in child psychology are similar. The first stages that unfold early in life are simple, and each subsequent stage builds on the earlier ones. What we observe as complex behaviors actually start out simple, but echo through subsequent development. In this way our psychological development mirrors our brain development.

Brain Development Begins as a Bounty of Opportunity

The power of a brain is directly related to the number of cells it has. The great evolutionary success of the human species has to do with our large number of brain cells and the connections among them. In only thirty-six hours of embryonic development the human brain produces several times as many cells as are found in a monkey's brain.[1]

During fetal life, the brain produces brain cells and connections in great abundance, actually twice as many as needed for postnatal life. These cells then compete to connect with a functioning part of the fetal body. Once connected, the body provides chemical feedback that segregates the cells with similar functions and connections into functional units. They in turn grow connections among themselves and start sending impulses together.

This organized firing of brain cells is not random, but it is far from predetermined. As the cells fire together, the connections among the nerve cells and the nerve fiber trunks grow stronger. In the beginning the response might be more random, and with time become more specific as the trunks of nerves are better defined with use. The cells that fire together stay together and recruit more nerve cells. Those that fail to fire, or get connected, or receive proper feedback from the body's organs, die.[2]

This is the way the brain organizes itself around body functions. If there is a limitation in the function of an organ like a muscle group in a limb, the brain does not develop properly. Proper body functions determine the form of the brain.

Halfway through fetal life, brain cells start to die, while others make more connections with their neighbors. Each fetus builds a brain with a unique organization. Like our fingerprints, no two brains are alike, not even in identical twins. Our brain, our personality, and our intelligence are all products of an elaborate interplay of intrauterine nurture and genetic heritage.

This complex process leaves humans with 200 billion brain cells at birth, putting the human species in its own class. Only humans have self-awareness, control over emotions, language, and abstract thinking—all qualities that are unparalleled in the universe.

The massive proliferation of connections among brain cells happens at an enormous speed. But this wiring process of the brain does not stop with the infant's birth. It continues until just before puberty, when there is another severe cropping of nerve connections. The ones not used are severed. Childhood stress and/or lack of stimulation can adversely affect these early growth spurts and alter how the nerve networks develop. From birth to twelve years the number of connections could vary as much as 25 percent depending on whether the child grows in an enriched or impoverished environment.

At birth the human brain weighs only 25 percent of its eventual adult weight. Our closest primate relative, the chimpanzee, is born with 45 percent of his adult brain weight already developed, and his brain growth slows down shortly after birth while the human brain growth continues at the fetal rate for the first two years of life. An infant brain's metabolic rate during his first two years is three times that of an adult. Then between two and ten years of age, the metabolic rate slows to twice that of an adult, and then begins to slow down until puberty, when the brain finishes its maturation.[3]

These startling facts mean that three fourths of human brain growth is after birth when the infant directly relates to his environment. During this time of rapid growth the brain is constantly making or breaking the connections between nerve cells and eagerly seeks information from the senses in redesigning its architecture. After age twelve, the nerve maps are set, which makes learning new skills difficult.[4]

In Early Neurodevelopment, Form Follows Function

The fetal brain's first goal is to control its developing body. The nerve cells in the central nervous system send their fibers out into the body to control its movement and structure and to receive information back into the brain. Brain sculpting in fetal life is driven by the function of the organs connected to the nervous system. Body movements and sensory input help the brain self-organize its wiring. The ability of nerve cells to change function was well illustrated in a monkey experiment where one finger was immobilized long enough for the monkey to lose function in the digit. When the monkey's brain was examined, it was discovered that the neurons that had controlled the restricted finger had switched their allegiance to controlling the functioning parts of the hand.[5] A fetus starts moving his limbs at seven weeks after conception. This activity is important in the neurodevelopment of the motor system. The nerves from the spinal cord link up with the muscles, but if the normal progression of the process is interrupted, the muscle cells start sending out messages to attract other nerve fibers. The nerves find the muscle fibers like salmon returning from the ocean to find their place of birth miles up stream.

The exact mechanisms of the self-organization that lead to fetal behavioral patterns are not fully understood, but neuroscientists are confident that later behavioral patterns build on the ones developed early in gestation. As the unborn child becomes more mature, so does his behavior. I watch in amazement as my tiny patients learn to recognize the difference between me and their parents. I now tell all my patients, including my most premature ones, that I am their doctor, so they will not equate the pain I must inflict on them at times with what their parents will do. Eventually they will react with stress behavior when I approach and with acute attentiveness when their parents approach. This happens within weeks of their birth and as early as twenty-seven to twenty-eight weeks' gestational age. To me, this is concrete evidence that the fetus has a memory and is capable of learning. He is also able to interact with adults in ways that capture our love and attentiveness.

This information emphasizes the importance of taking fetal love breaks frequently each day. Your fetal love messages teach your developing child to expect love from her environment. Her brain will organize itself around the anticipation of receiving love. Later in life as her brain and behaviors become more complex they will build on a foundation of love.

Let's Talk About Numbers

The adult brain has about 100 billion nerve cells—about the same number of stars in our galaxy, the Milky Way. At eighteen weeks of gestation there are about 200 billion nerve cells in the fetal brain. Their origin occurs deep in the center of the brain at the second stage of development, and then they migrate out in an orderly fashion to the cortex. The relative distance a nerve cell travels from where it germinates to its final resting place is about the same as us walking from New York to San Francisco. Each individual nerve cell makes this trek in a matter of weeks. At first, a series of scout cells moves toward the brain's cortex. They are then followed by the nerve cells (neurons). This occurs in waves of movement and each subsequent wave pushes beyond the last, bulging the brain cortex into the convolutions we see on the brain's surface.

Three critical phases occur in a nerve cell's development. They are born, they migrate to their proper place, and they begin to fire impulses that excite the nerves around them. Each phase in this development depends on the successful completion of the previous phase. So any small defect early in brain development will be magnified as fetal life continues. The birth of nerve cells and their disbursement toward their individual final resting places in the mature brain bears a close resemblance to the explosive dispersion of stars in the Big Bang that gave birth to the universe. Each cell must be in the correct place at the right time for this very complex developmental process to go smoothly.

As each wave of neurons passes the previous one, molecular information is exchanged and they make connections that are important in the coordination of later brain development. These connections can last a lifetime or fall apart soon after the early migration. Some of the known causes for problems during this critical phase of neuron birth and migration are not enough oxygen or glucose, or too much cortisol, alcohol, or exposure to neurotoxic drugs.

There is another system of cells in our brain that also develops along with the nerve cells. They are called glial cells and they also number about 100 billion in the adult brain. For proper brain function these cells must also reside in their proper location. The glial cells surround, protect, and nourish the nerve trunks that carry the nerve impulses. Once the glial cell insulates the cell's axon or trunk with myelin, the impulses travel at a faster rate.

At birth each neuron has about 2,500 connections, called synapses, with other nerve cells. These continue to increase until reaching a peak at eight months, when there are about 15,000 synapses per neuron. At this time the baby's brain has 1,000 trillion synapses. What a huge number. Here's a way you can get a handle on it. If an electrician was wiring a supercomputer with this many connections and he could make one connection a second, it would take him 30 million years to finish the job![6] That's a long time. To build his brain a man would have to start before he evolved from his prehistoric ancestors 200,000 years ago.

All of these brain cell connections give the infant and young child a great advantage in learning to adapt to his environment; but by the time he reaches his tenth birthday, the number of brain cell connections are reduced to 500 trillion through a process of pruning the inactive connections. What he does not use he loses.

This description of the astronomical numbers of cells and connections in the human brain falls short of quantifying the magnificence of this amazing organ. It is far more capable and complex than what we understand. I am sure as the neurosciences develop, we will learn many more impressive statistics about the brain.

4

$\mathcal{F}$etal Development of Senses

We live on the leash of our senses.

—*Diane Ackerman*

I am amazed at how early in gestation the fetus develops his senses. I used to wonder why they are there when he really has no use for them. But with more being learned about fetal development and behavior, I am confident that one day we will discover their importance. In this section I will describe each sense's development. I think you will also be amazed at your unborn child's neurological capacity.

Taste and Smell

The taste buds and olfactory bulb start developing at eight weeks and are mature and fully functional by fifteen weeks of gestation. No more development takes place after this time. They are anatomically just like yours and mine, but they are far more capable than any adult's. The senses of taste and smell are closely linked and are directly connected by large nerve tracks with the midbrain. This area of the brain also develops early in gestation and is the crucible for our emotions. Because it develops early in gestation, it is sensitive to sensory input during fetal life.

From this very young age, your unborn child prefers sweets. When glucose is placed in the amniotic fluid, the infant's swallowing activity increases significantly. After birth, most full-term infants will crawl up their mother's abdomen and chest to start sucking at her breasts. The infant is guided to his mother's breasts by their smell. Around the mother's nipples are small glands that secrete a lipid that smells and tastes like her amniotic fluid, which the fetus has been tasting for months. I also think the sucking and swallowing are reinforced by the milk's sweet taste.

For our sick, very preterm infants, we dip small cotton sticks in their mother's breast milk and let them suck on it like a pacifier. This usually settles an agitated infant, and primes the intestinal track for digesting the small amounts of breast milk we give him. We usually start a premature infant on four to five drops of breast milk every three to six hours. This relaxes him and gives him a sense of peace.

After birth, a full-term infant learns quickly to differentiate his mother's milk from other breast milk. When I smell breast milk, I can't discern any difference in the samples from different mothers, but a six-week-old term infant can smell his mother as soon as she opens the front door of their home. Partners report different behaviors of newborns when their spouses enter the house.

It is a good idea to use this exquisite sense of smell as a psychological tool for emotional attachment between you and your child. If you decide to breast-feed your infant and have to leave her, I suggest you place your used lactating pads or a worn bra in the infant's room as an odor reminder of your presence. Mothers also have an armpit signature that infants easily recognize.

Infants' sense of smell is so keen that they can discern odors in combination with others, and can select the pleasant odors in the presence of others. This is a highly developed skill, but how an infant learns strong preferences without previous extrauterine experience is unknown. We adults certainly do not have this capability. We have lost our sense of smell from disuse!

Touch

The next sense to be developed in the fetus is touch, which is present sixteen weeks after conception. Touch is perceived by us in the cortex, but the nerve impulses from the touch receptors in the skin pass through the midbrain before reaching the cortex. This is why touch can be filled with so many emotional overtones. At twenty-three to twenty-seven weeks of gestation, touch is fully developed. I frequently use it to console my agitated patients. Pregnant mothers also rub their abdomens from about twenty-three weeks until they deliver, and most tell me they do this because it comforts their unborn child. Abdominal rubbing can console the active baby who is kicking in utero. Try it and see what happens. This fetal love message teaches your unborn child that she has some control over your availability to console her. This is the inception of her emerging self-esteem.

Tiffany Fields at the University of Florida has shown that massage therapy for patients in the intensive care nursery increases the premature infants' rate of weight gain and allows them to go home at an earlier age.[1] In India, Mother Teresa used infant massage and frequently extolled its benefits to critically ill infants.

In our nursery we use a technique called "kangaroo care," where we place our patients skin-to-skin on the chest of his mother or father sitting in a rocking chair. They are then wrapped together with a blanket to keep the infant warm. I have done this with my sickest patients, and I have watched in amazement as the infant's heart rate, blood pressure, and blood oxygen tension all improve. Many times I ask the couple to either talk in quiet tones or to sing and play music while they give kangaroo care. I have seen many infants at twenty-eight weeks smile serenely with their eyes while receiving this loving attention. It is extremely enjoyable for both parent and patient.

Sight

There are many misconceptions among my colleagues about a newborn's vision. You've probably seen black-and-white mobiles or other objects for a newborn's crib. It is a mistake to use only black and white, because there is definite evidence that newborns can see colors and are more interested in them. They even can discern colors of different hues, which implies remarkable maturity of the visual cortex.

Robert Fantz at Case Western Reserve University watched newborn eye movements through a peephole and was able to tell how long and at what they were looking by the reflections off the eye's cornea.

He has demonstrated that newborn infants prefer patterns, curves, colors, drawings in three dimensions, and faces. They have depth perception and will reach out if properly supported. Their reach appears to be limited more by their neuromuscular control of their hand and arm than by their eye-hand coordination. In the past clinicians evaluated neurodevelopment and health of newborns' nervous systems by the infants' neuromuscular abilities, but now we know there is much more going on in their brains, which is limited by their immature neuromuscular development.[2]

Tom Bower at University of Edinburgh showed head movement and eye widening when an object was moved toward a newborn's face. This demonstrated the baby's ability to perceive three dimensions and to coordinate what was seen with the muscles that moved his head in order to avoid the object coming toward his face. When objects appear as illusions with the use of polarizing goggles and filters, the infants reached out to touch the illusion and when they could not make contact with their hands, they reacted with scowls on their faces.[3]

I have observed that when the hands of a term infant touch an unnoticed ball by random movements, his eyes will immediately look right at the ball. This extremely sophisticated spatial perception and coordination between his vision and the rest of his body was all developed in utero.

To me the most amazing visual ability of the newborn is his eagerness to look at human faces right after birth. One can show newborns all types of pictures and designs, but a human face always draws more attention. This is apparent even right after birth, before the newborn knows what a human face looks like. Within hours he is able to pick out a picture of his mother's face when lined up with several other faces of adult females. This is an example not only of his visual acuity but also of the quickness of his memory.

When I look into the face of a healthy newborn, it appears that I have his undivided attention. His eyes are fixed right into the center of my forehead. They are looking more at my eyes than at my mouth, but I have seen him reflect my smile with a very subtle "smile" in his eyes. Watch your newborn's eyes. You will soon learn to read his moods and interests.

If you want to show your newborn infant something, hold it about two feet from his face. That is where his eyes focus best and, interestingly, is the distance between the faces of a newborn and his mother while breastfeeding. I also suggest you decorate his crib and mobiles with pictures of you and your husband rather than nursery rhyme characters. If you don't have pictures, then draw "smiley faces" on bright stickers and place them around the crib's bumper. Be sure to use vivid, high-contrast colors.

Hearing

The cochlea (the part of the ear that changes sound into nerve impulses) with its nerve pathways is well developed by twenty weeks of fetal life. This trunk of nerves is one of the earliest to fully develop, as are the nerves that interpret the sounds. At twenty-two weeks of gestation the developing infant will respond to sounds from outside the womb. By twenty-eight weeks the infant responds to sound in very consistent ways.

Each of the other senses has specific parts of the brain in which it develops, while hearing and speech can develop in nearly any area of the brain's cortex. The speech area is usually in the left or dominant hemisphere of the brain, but in some right-handed people it develops in the right hemisphere. If the speech area of the brain is damaged, it can then develop in a different part of the cortex. Language is so important to the brain that it will not let it go. And certainly speech is one of the distinguishing attributes of being human.[4]

The fetus may not hear with his ears alone. His entire body may resonate with the sounds that surround him. There are many examples of deaf people learning to perceive sound using other senses. Helen Keller was both blind and deaf, but she learned to hear through her hands. Beethoven was deaf by the time he wrote and conducted his last major works. Plants obviously don't have ears, yet they respond to music. Most houseplants grow faster and flower more with classical music rather than hard rock music. Even inert bodies resonate with sound. For example, a note struck on a piano in a room filled with pianos will sound different because the same note on all the other pianos, as well as others in the harmonic series (overtones) will vibrate in harmony.

A baby's auditory perceptual field at birth is able to distinguish all different speech sounds in all the world languages, but he unfortunately loses this ability by age one. Different languages have different auditory maps, and after his first year, the child can no longer distinguish the subtle differences in the sounds of languages different from the native one he has heard since before his birth. By age ten, a child can't learn to speak a foreign language without an accent.

I have taught prenatal classes to pregnant parents for decades, and I encourage them to read aloud, or play and sing their favorite inspirational music, which relaxes both parents and their unborn child. Later, when the parents are having difficulty quieting the child, I suggest they play the same music they did during the pregnancy. The child's response is almost immediate and she usually stops crying. The musical fetal love message conditioned her to relax like her mother did when they both heard the parents' favorite music.

I can always tell which of my full-term newborn infants have been read to. They have more mature orienting behavior to auditory stimuli. I can even tell which fathers have been active in reading to their unborn child. I do this by holding the infant between me and his father while we compete for the infant's attention by calling the child's name. If the dad has been actively involved in the reading and singing, his child will turn his head toward him, looking for the source of the sound. Invariably, when their eyes meet they both react positively.

Because infants before birth favor higher-pitched sounds, fathers who want to communicate with their unborn child need to get close and raise the pitch of their voice. Mothers seem to know this instinctively. They speak to their infant in a special language called "motherese," which seems to greatly stimulate the nervous system. Their voice pitch, rhythm, and tones are involuntarily set to stimulate their infant's brain with maximum effect.

Within weeks of birth, term infants are able to discern when lip movements fit the sounds they are hearing. If the mother's voice is presented along with someone else's face, the newborn becomes disturbed and turns his head away from the face and sound, showing a primitive form of lipreading while face-to-face with the speaker.

Dr. Henry Truby reports that infants have similar "crying patterns" to their parents' speech patterns and believes that infants not only hear in utero, but also practice the mouth and breathing movements of speech and crying. He has studied the sound waves of infant's cries and calls these patterns "cryprints." He has found the "cryprints" of even a premature infant to be the same as his parents'. The fetus is taking language lessons from his mother as early as twenty-eight weeks! If his mother is mute, the cry of the newborn infant is different right from birth, revealing that he has missed an auditory experience in utero.[5] Normal babies are disturbed by other babies' crying. The effect is even greater the closer they are in age, which implies that crying is communication to other babies. When a baby hears a recording of his own cry he gets very upset, and infants in a nursery with a crying baby will cry more than in a quiet nursery.

Auditory Environment

The fetal environment is rich in auditory stimulation, which includes the mother's pulse, her intestinal gurgles, her breathing, and—with remarkable clarity—her voice. The loudest of these is the intestinal noise. Then comes the sound of her blood pulsing through the uterine vessels. This has been demonstrated both in animals and in humans who were in labor with a small microphone placed in the uterine cavity after the fetal membranes ruptured when the water broke. These data clearly demonstrate that the mother's voice is distinct and can easily be heard.

The fetal experience with his mother's voice is important in a child's early social process as well as in his later emotional development. If the mother's voice is shrill or alarming or angry, Dr. Tomatis has found the preborn learns to dread it and will have a reaction different from the eager searching for contact with the speaker that most babies demonstrate after birth.

Premature infants have neural and cardiac responses to noise as early as twenty-four weeks after conception. By twenty-eight to twenty-nine weeks they can distinguish other voices from their mother's. There is no reason for me to think that intrauterine auditory development is any different from this extrauterine development, so the fetus hears and learns from what his parents are saying to him and to each other. We'll talk about this important fact some more in later chapters.

The sound of the mother's pulse is also important to the unborn child's development both physically and psychologically. Psychologist Lee Salk reports that 80 percent of paintings of a madonna show her holding the infant's head toward her left side or over her heart. Using heart sounds in the nursery, Dr. Salk was able to get babies to grow faster, sleep better, and cry less. The heartbeat had to be 72 beats per minute. One that was 128 beats per minute irritated the infants, and the researchers had to stop the experiment because of the adverse reactions. Again these data illustrate the importance of the fetal love breaks and learning how to reduce anxiety and safely express your negative emotions. Have you ever wondered how much your unborn child knows about you? Keep reading.

$\mathcal{T}$he Intrauterine Temple of Learning

Knowledge is the mother of all virtue, all vice proceeds from ignorance.

—Proverbs

As you've already become very aware, now is the time you most affect your baby's future. Think way into the future, to when your child is an adult finishing his formal education and starting his own family. Think about what kind of student, spouse, parent, and worker you want him to be. You need to decide now, because the brain he needs to reach those goals is developing now—in utero. During childhood his brain architecture can change, but the older the brain becomes the more difficult change becomes. There is no better time to shape his behavior and temperament than now and shortly after his birth.

Some parents think they need to develop an educational system like flash cards or send their infants to "better baby institutes" to properly stimulate their infant's brain. All of this is not necessary. The baby is equipped to learn all he needs to learn from playing and interacting with the people who love him. The most important advice I can give you is to take the time and energy to use your natural ability in helping babies learn. Nature designed you to teach babies. Babies are designed to learn from you. This adage is just as true before birth.

It is incorrect to think unborn children have no ability in higher brain function. Brain activity starts six weeks after conception. At eight weeks the fetus extends his arm and shoulder and flexes his back to push away from a fine hair brushing his cheek. Mothers don't report movements until twenty weeks, but the uterus is insensitive to touch, so fetal movements must stretch the uterus for the mother to feel them.

At fourteen weeks he has facial expressions. Brain wave tests show that the fetus's brain cortex is working at twenty-eight weeks. The brain waves also prove that the cortex receives impulses from vision, touch, and hearing and he can respond meaningfully to these sensory experiences at twenty-eight weeks. From thirty-two weeks your infant responds to your movements and tries to stabilize himself by waving his arms and legs. Dutch scientists describe these exercises as graceful, voluntary, and spontaneous.[1]

Perinatologists report that fetuses try to avoid the needles they insert into the uterine cavity for sampling amniotic fluid or fetal blood. They have purposeful movements with their arms and feet. These movements are better coordinated and appear more mature than the ones I am able to watch in my tiny patients who are stressed and lose their coordination. My patients are stressed and their brains disorganize quickly after a premature birth.

The Emotional Characteristics of a Successful Adult

Modern psychology and the business world are beginning to appreciate that there is more to success than academic performance. A brilliant scholar may not be successful in the business world because he lacks the emotional skills that are needed for effective communication and leadership. On the other hand, an effective communicator, perhaps not as intelligent as the scholar, but someone who can organize and motivate a workforce, is a great asset and may be more successful in a corporation than the scholar.

To have a successful marriage and to raise children properly, we all need control over our emotional impulses. Aristotle, the great Greek educator, stated it well in the *Nicomachean Ethics;* "Anyone can become angry, that is easy. But to be angry with the right person, to the right degree, at the right time, for the right purpose, and in the right way, this is not easy."

As businesses begin to divide their missions into smaller and smaller components that are assigned to small action groups of workers, the ability to effectively communicate, lead, and motivate becomes more important than the employee's ability to understand all the technical information about the business. The types of interpersonal and communication skills that serve adults well are learned in early childhood. Colleges and numerous postgraduate courses try to teach them, but they are far more easily learned and practiced in early infancy.

I repeat, now is the time to think about what gifts (the ones money cannot buy) you want to give your unborn child, and start doing the important work to ensure they have them later. Please review your sentence stems from chapter 1. After learning this important information about intrauterine brain development you probably want to add more endings to your sentence stems.

Psychologists have divided our personal power into two basic components. One is the old standard of intelligence as measured by IQ tests and academic performance. The other, which is emerging as equally important, is a measure of emotional competence called the "emotional quotient." We need both in order to be successful in all aspects of our lives, to be educated, and to have emotional maturity.[2]

You have the opportunity to give both of these "quotient gifts" to your unborn and newly born child. And I emphasize both—otherwise how can we explain that some people with high intelligence are not successful while others with modest intellect are extremely successful in all aspects of adult life?

Most "successful" people have qualities that helped them achieve their success. These include, among others, high self-esteem, zeal, self-control, persistence, and self-motivation. America has a list of presidents who were not exactly geniuses but were highly effective because of their ability to communicate and motivate people.

Unfortunately, most parents are very concerned about their child's intellectual development, but miss important opportunities to help their child build a competent brain because they wait too long to take action. They have the misconception that neurodevelopment during the period of intrauterine life and first few years after birth are not as important as when their child starts preschool. For years medical science aided and abetted these misguided parents by fostering the perception that a child's brain must unfold along a genetic timetable and that early stimulation did not improve later academic performance.

Unfortunately, scientists were using the wrong stimulation to get the expected results. It is fruitless to bring to an infant the teaching techniques designed for a three-year-old. They will not work, but that does not mean the infant's brain is unable to learn. There is no time in a person's life when more can be done for intellectual prowess than when his brain is developing. Your unborn infant's brain is a dynamic and powerful organ with incredible flexibility, or brain plasticity, which allows the brain to adapt quickly and easily to its environment.

The periods of active development that occur in utero and for the first two years after birth are called "critical periods" or windows of time when a specific part of the brain is receptive to growth and change. During a critical period, brain development depends on proper stimulation. If the proper stimulus occurs after the critical period closes, brain growth may not proceed. Fortunately, the boundaries of critical periods are soft, and after they close, all hope is not lost, but the neurodevelopment takes much more effort. Adults have passed many critical periods, but we are still able to learn new skills. It just takes us longer and requires more effort than for our children. Vision and language development are classic examples of critical periods.[3]

Here's an interesting example. Dr. David Hubel and Dorsten Wiesel won a Nobel Prize for research done forty years ago that demonstrated the importance of the critical period, using cats as a model. They sewed shut one eye of a newborn kitten to test the effect of sensory deprivation. When the shut eye was opened a few weeks later, the cat was permanently blinded. There was nothing anatomically wrong with the cat's eye. The lack of stimulation during a critical period of brain development caused the blindness in the visual cortex of the cat's developing brain.

Interestingly, the eye that remained open had better visual acuity than normal cat eyes. However, no amount of visual stimulation could restore sight in the closed eye after the critical period had passed. Thus we learned that sensory input is essential for brain development.[4]

Babies with cataracts who don't receive surgery to remove them in the first couple of months after birth will permanently lose their vision, and again, no stimulation after the cataract removal will restore the blind child's vision. A baby deprived of vision for just four months will remain blind for the rest of his life.

Here are a few examples of how you can stimulate your unborn child's brain development. After twenty-three weeks of pregnancy you can soothe her by rubbing your uterus. When you have an unsettling experience, the kind we all have every day, take time to recover from the event psychologically and spiritually as described in the book's later chapters. For now you have enough information to take a fetal love break when stressed. Play music that relaxes you and rub your abdomen. Later you will read about using your brain to send chemical fetal love messages to your unborn child.

Prenatal Intellectual Development

Fetuses and newborn infants should be living in very enriched environments. I'm sure you want to make your child's brain crackle with synaptic activity, since his nerve cells require proper stimulation to grow and develop. At the simplest level, a neuron in a culture dish will grow better and make more connections with its neighboring cells if stimulated with an electrical impulse. In the developing central nervous system, nerve cells that are active release growth factors that stimulate other nerve cells to connect with them. The more a pathway is stimulated, the more connections it makes with other neurons, and the thicker and more permanent they become.

Rats raised in a rich environment, with wheels to spin, ladders to climb, and other rats as playmates had thicker brains, 25 percent more connections between nerve cells, and were smarter than rats raised with no cage mates or toys. Both groups were given the same amount and type of food. Amazingly, this effect was passed on to the next generation of rats. Pregnant rats in an enriched environment produced newborn rats with thicker cortexes than those that lived in the impoverished environment. This experiment did not produce supersmart rats but rather showed the effects an impoverished environment has on brain growth both prenatally and postnatally.

Dr. Craig Ramey at the University of Alabama found he could produce the same results in children. He took a group of impoverished inner-city children whose mothers had IQs less than 70. At age four months he split the infants into two groups. One acted as a control where there was no intervention. The second group was exposed daily to an enriched environment of learning with toys and playmates (similar to the rats' enriched environment). At age three the stimulated group of children had an average of 20 IQ points higher than the control group of children, who all emerged in grade school retarded or with borderline intelligence. When the children did not get intervention until age five, 86 percent of them tested with IQs below 85.

When he tested the experimental group's IQs twelve years later, he found they had maintained their higher IQ scores; their brains were more active, as determined by PET scans, which measure the brain's metabolic activity; and they were doing better in school than the children from the same background but without the advantage of the enriched environment. Dr. Ramey states, "In at least eleven separate studies, we have data to show that, if you don't intervene before twenty-four months, these children will be seriously developmentally delayed. And, we have no data to show that we can reverse the majority of these delays."[5]

For years psychologists and sociologists have thought the IQ of the infant's mother was the strongest predictor of a child's IQ. They are correct, but their reason for the association was incorrect, and it stifled research in this area for years. They thought the effect was simply genetics and early intervention would not work. Now Dr. Ramsey has shown clearly that intervention works, and the earlier it starts, the better the results. In fact, he concludes that the effect of poor stimulation on brain structure may be so great that it is not correctable after age five.

In a similar study of four-month-old babies whose mothers engaged them in ways that provided them opportunities to observe, imitate, and learn, the children performed higher on IQ tests at age four than children who did not get the same teaching until eight months later at age one. The authors concluded that the earlier the intervention, the larger the effect.

I absolutely believe this to be true and that is why I am encouraging you to start stimulating your unborn child now! If nothing else, consider the following experiment.

Anthony Casper at the University of North Carolina had pregnant mothers read aloud the popular Dr. Seuss book *The Cat in the Hat* twice a day to their unborn children. A few days after birth the newborns were given the opportunity to hear another Dr. Seuss story. The infants were outfitted with a special nipple that let them change the story read by altering the speed of their sucking.

As demonstrated by their sucking speed, the newborns remembered *The Cat in the Hat,* liked it better than the new story, and adjusted their sucking speed to hear the familiar one. They preferred the story read by their mother over another female reader. Furthermore, they preferred it read forward instead of backward.[6] Amazing!

Babies learn by imitation, which is uniquely human. Not only do babies imitate adults, but adults imitate babies. Watch a mother feeding a baby: she opens her mouth as she brings the food up to the baby's mouth. Babies know when adults are imitating them and they like it. By imitating their parents' behaviors, babies learn how to function in the culture around them. This is why human contact is so vital for normal baby development. They need face-to-face contact to watch the facial expressions. Using the combination of imitating their infants and speaking "motherese," mothers naturally stimulate brain development in their infants.

Parents hear so much about the devastating effect of poor nutrition on children's mental development. It is true that good nutrition helps your child build good immunity to prevent infections and is needed for growth, but the brain's "food" is education and it thrives on stimulation.

How rich this banquet is affects how well brains grow and develop. I liken a parent's work with her unborn child to that of a farmer in his vineyard who prunes his grapevines so some branches get stronger and produce more fruit. With proper cultivation, your infant's brain, like the farmer's fruit, will provide a bountiful harvest. The brain makes the active synapses stronger by pruning the ones not in use. It basically saves the circuits that experience has shown to be useful, and crops the rest.

Humans are designed for communication. Infants come into the world prepared to participate in this exchange. They need constant contact with caregivers. Without it, development goes awry. The communication between parent and infant is a vital nutrient for a growing brain. Babies want and deserve to be the center of our world. The best way to enrich your unborn child's intellectual environment is constantly to talk and sing to him. Words are like little carpenters that enter the brain to build the centers dedicated to receptive and expressive language. Exposure to human speech builds circuitry in the brain that allows more words to be absorbed. Children whose mothers talk with them frequently have better language skills than children whose mothers seldom do. This effect is similar to the one described previously with the use of music to help stimulate the part of the brain that deals with math concepts and spatial reasoning.

Recent research data lead developmental psychologists to conclude that babies are just plain smarter than we are. Infant brains are better at learning, because they have more nerve cells with more connections among them, which makes it easier for them to learn something new. The advantage we have over them is that we were once babies and have already gone through the learning process and have our brains well tuned to our environment. We adults can make some minor improvements in our knowledge and skill levels, but it sure is easier at an earlier age.[7]

6

$\mathcal{I}$ntrauterine Emotional Development

Life without emotion is like an engine without fuel.

—*Mary Astor*

Today there is anatomical evidence that the brain centers that affect our behaviors develop before birth. My colleagues and I see sophisticated behaviors develop in premature infants every day. The same behavioral development we observe occurs in the baby you are gestating. Because of my experience in observing premature infants' development, I know your baby well. During the later stages of your pregnancy, I can tell you about the development of your baby's behavior week by week.

I also know about organ development during fetal gestation. Each organ goes through a critical period of development when the number of its cells has reached a critical level and the organ is ready to start its mature function. The acquisition of mature function in a fetal organ is called the critical period of development. It is similar to maturational changes that occur as our children go through puberty, but the changes in utero are more dramatic.

Psychologists use the concept of critical periods also in children's psychological development. They rename them "sensitive periods" because their boundaries are not as well defined as the critical periods of neurodevelopment. The tragic aspect of these two periods in development is that they occur early in life and once past, developmental problems are difficult to correct. Most researchers think that some early experiences cannot be undone. If a child does not get the proper emotional stimulation during a sensitive period, then his ability to develop the quality may be lost forever. If he does not learn to monitor and control his emotions during a sensitive period early in life, he may never learn how to do it and will grow up being impulsive. Later in life, with psychotherapy, he may be able control his impulsive outbursts, but certainly it is much harder to do. If a child lacks exposure to parental contact and trust during the important development stage, then as an adult he may not develop the behaviors of spontaneous affection and trust in relationships.

Psychologists accept the concept that early childhood experiences affect our mental health and intelligence as adults, but few are willing to consider prenatal events as being as important. I don't understand or agree with their lack of interest in the prenatal environment, since the brain passes through many more critical periods of development prenatally than after birth. But since it is only recently that we have the sophisticated instruments and techniques to observe and study the fetus, I think neuroscientists and psychologists were limited by poor access to the unborn child.

The developing brain is exposed to two environments—one in utero and the other after birth. The main difference between the two is the effect a mother has on the environments. Inside the womb, the infant indirectly experiences his mother's external circumstances. In addition, his brain is washed by neuropeptides (more about these molecules of emotion later) that reflect his mother's emotional reactions to the external environment. Your baby's brain is being conditioned by your every reaction to your life situation and changing environments.

This intrauterine experience prepares the unborn infant for his birth environment. And his emotional education continues outside the womb when the infant observes and learns from his mother's behaviors and facial expressions.

An example of the power of intrauterine learning was demonstrated in a study looking at what changes occur in fetal behavior with maternal smoking. When a mother smokes, her fetus responds with heaving respiratory movements and an accelerated heart rate—the way we adults respond to the sudden drop in our blood oxygen content when a plastic bag is placed over our head. By six months' gestation, when learning and memory are present, the fetus's heart rate increases and he starts gasping when his mother just thinks about smoking.[1]

This study clearly demonstrates that the unborn infant has a memory and experiences his mother's cravings. It also is a graphic example of how harmful smoking is to the unborn child. Most mothers who smoke would never suffocate their newborn infant. They just are not fully aware of how uncomfortable their smoking is to their developing fetus.

The use of street drugs probably has the same devastating effect on the emotional well-being of the unborn child, who shares her mother's drug addiction and withdrawal symptoms. Neonatologists constantly see this behavior in infants delivered by mothers using illicit drugs. It is not pleasant when we have to give our newborn patient the same addicting drug or a similar one and then slowly withdraw it over weeks to months. The addicted baby cannot sleep, constantly cries, is easily startled, has difficulty eating, and may die. After her birth we can monitor her behavior. However, in utero there is no way to monitor adequately the same severe drug withdrawal symptoms.

Let's return now to those neuropeptides I mentioned. There is no other time in your child's life when you have as much influence over his emotional development as during pregnancy. You and your unborn infant are connected in a most intimate way by the passage of neuropeptides across the placenta. These powerful molecules affect your unborn child's prenatal emotional development by altering brain structure and setting his own neuropeptide concentrations. The behavior we see in our newborn infants is not simply a genetic expression; it is a combination of genetic expression and fetal experience. As the fetus progresses through its prenatal psychological development, the variety of behaviors narrows. Once an unborn child starts along a path of behavioral development, it becomes harder to change.

Let's look at a powerful example. The child listens in on a conversation between his mother and father. The conversation is about a joyful memory of a pleasant experience in the recent past. The infant's mother is enjoying her partner's rendition of what happened and her brain is secreting neuropeptides that make her feel content, loved, and safe. Soon she's flush with laughter and love for the father of her unborn child.

The neuropeptides produced by her brain flow out into the bloodstream and cross the placenta to bathe the developing baby's brain. The infant's brain is affected by this experience and after twenty-eight weeks of pregnancy he will remember the emotions he passively experienced while hearing his parents' laughter and conversation. This is the beginning of the child's emotional development and, like the other aspects of brain formation, the early simple experiences are the foundations for later reactions to similar stimuli. This is how your infant prepares for the emotional world he will greet after birth.

Now consider another example of a pregnant couple whose relationship is not as loving. Let's say the mother's life partner is ridiculing her and using laughter as a tool to demean and intimidate her. The mixture of neuropeptides will be totally different and the unborn's brain will receive an entirely different message from his mother's neuropeptide mix. A different memory is formed and a different expectation is carried forward. After birth this child will respond to his father's laughter differently. His expectations about his environment have been set by the neuropeptide mix that his mother had during the incident of ridiculing laughter.

The baby in our first example will expect love and attention, while the other will anticipate anxiety and insecurity when his father laughs. That is why it is so important to work on the exercises presented in part 3 of this book on how to control your emotions and to relate effectively to your partner.

For a permanent effect on a newborn's behavior, the unborn child needs long and frequent exposure to a particular set of neuropeptides. Unfortunately, we in medicine know more about the negative effects of stress neuropeptides than we do about the ones associated with positive emotions.

Parents usually tend to focus more on intellectual capacities and don't ask about their children's emotional development and adult emotional health. In my opinion, the latter is far more important to society and to the overall success of their adult child than his IQ.

Let's review. From midgestation until two years after birth, your child develops a template of expectations about himself and the world around him. This is the foundation of who he becomes and how he relates to others. A child's personality is in place long before he enters preschool. Psychologists tell us they can recognize which children are going to get into trouble in their teenage years by the time they are two years old.[2] They also state that the earlier therapeutic intervention occurs, the more likely it is to be successful. The critical period for emotional development is just before birth and for the next two years. After that time, a kind of permanence or irreversibility sets in, and from then on the brain design is not going to change very much.

Early infancy is the time when children learn empathy, emotional attachment to others, and how to control and balance feelings. If a child experiences love he will learn to expect it when approaching new situations.

The biology of our species makes it mandatory for a huge investment in parenting to achieve the fulfillment of a child's potential. A Yale University neurobiologist, Dr. Mathma Constantine Paton, stated it well: "Such knowledge provides the moral and social imperative to prevent or cure brain damage caused by the lack of proper environmental stimulation during the brain's crucial period of development in fetal life and childhood." There is no better or more important gift to your child or society.

A healthy early relationship between parent and infant is one that allows the infant to freely express his emotions with the expectation that he will quickly be soothed and comforted. This is a fluid exchange of emotional energy between parent and child.

There is a time for giving and a time for receiving, both more of an attitude than a skill. Every interchange you have with your child is a magic moment to shape the child's brain, to hurt or to build. Even tiny interactions between parent and infant are the building blocks of how well the child will function in the future. Each magic moment is another stitch in the tapestry that, when finished one day, will be the child's view of his world.

Here is a touching quest story of a close personal friend. I'm sure you'll note several important junctures that could have created a vastly different outcome for this child and his family.

Dick was a firstborn son with aggressive behavior at birth. I remember visiting his mother in the hospital when the nurse brought Dick into her room. He had cried most of the morning and was disturbing the nurses and other babies in the nursery.

As a toddler, Dick needed lots of stimulation to stay happy. If left alone he was soon bored and cried for stimulation. This was exhausting.

He stayed awake nights and obviously so did his dad and mother. After Dick's birth his dad had allowed him to cry, thinking that it would help him learn not to do it. I had been taught that too. We were wrong. Now I understand the neurochemical mechanisms that support the reasons why parents should respond quickly to crying children.

Dick's mother had a major life tragedy while she was pregnant with him. Both her parents died within three months of each other, and she was moved to a strange city, where she knew no one, so her husband could continue his education. She was left alone to mourn the tragic loss of both parents.

All through his young life Dick's parents tried to learn ways of keeping him contented, but it was impossible. He needed constant attention, which was not always available. His father was in his neonatal fellowship with me and then started a very busy practice. Dick was a challenge for preschool educators and for early grammar school teachers. He tested above normal in intelligence, but was impulsive. He progressed through school with just enough work to get by, but was by no means a good student. He had terrible work and study habits. His lack of school performance was a disappointment to both his parents.

Throughout his life he enjoyed stimulating activities like competitive sports and fast amusement park rides. His father had long talks with him about risk taking and his need to always face danger. But Dick liked the exhilarating feeling of facing danger, and this need to be stimulated by danger led him into dangerous sports like extreme skiing. Fortunately his coordination was excellent and he excelled in all sports.

I remember a conversation with Dick's mother when I told her that she had to let Dick find his own way of meeting his need for excitement. His temperament demanded it, and there was no way to control it, I said. I predicted he would die a violent death, but I hoped and prayed that he would live a long life. I knew he would eventually have become a productive adult because he was so well loved by many friends.

Dick died in an automobile accident at age twenty.

Looking back on his life, his dad told me that there were many things he wished he had done differently. I reminded him that at the time he was doing his best to love Dick with all his heart, knowledge, and talent. Obviously it was not enough. Dick's father could have been a better nest builder for his wife while she was pregnant with Dick. He was too busy and too self-absorbed with his work during his fellowship, plus he firmly believed that a father's role was to be the provider of financial security and not necessarily a nurturer of infants.

This was particularly true in the prenatal period. At the time of Dick's birth medical science had no concept about the prenatal development of psychological traits such as temperament. Now Dick's dad wishes he had the knowledge we have today, because he's sure he could have done things differently for his wife while she was carrying Dick and during the first two years of his life after birth. Dick would have been a happier child and his untimely death might have been prevented. My experience with Dick and his parents led me to the important conclusion that parenting children starts before birth. If Dick's parents knew how to give their developing child unconditional love before birth like they did after his birth, I now know his life would have been different.

The main job of an infant's brain is to figure out what kind of environment it lives in and to discover what responses improves his chances of survival. The newborn does this rapidly and is continually looking for feedback. If aggression is needed, then—from the trillions of connections in the brain—the ones reinforced are the aggressive ones that set his temperament and how he will react to stimuli. These environmentally induced brain changes can become permanent and literally code the genes for aggression and violence for a lifetime.

When children are delivered into a terrible environment and still do well, there is usually someone in their lives who instilled the concept that they are not helpless and they can do something to improve the situation.

And when children of good parents go bad there is a reason. At the University of Chicago neuroscientists have tracked down the environmental inputs that lead children to violence and aggression. Overwhelmingly it is stress. When kids are raised in violent, unsafe environments over which they have no control, they develop a stress-weary brain. These children need someone who makes them feel safe, gives them a feeling of self-worth, and teaches them their lives are not hopeless.

When a mother holds and cuddles her newborn infant, the baby's natural opiates are secreted from the base of the brain. This biologically builds the maternal-infant bond and the attachment process to a reward system of contentment.

This has been studied in monkeys by Dr. Gary Kraemer at the Harlow Primate Laboratory. Deprivation of adequate nurturing in the early life of infant monkeys led to dysregulation of their neurobiological process. The deprived monkeys either exaggerated or blunted their emotional responses and all had poor performances of cognitive tasks as adults. They were at risk for aggressive behaviors. When stressed as adults, they became over- or underresponsive, and their responses were unpredictable. Dr. Kraemer attributed this to the dysregulation of their brain neurotransmitters, which was set up by poor nurturing early in infancy.[3]

When an infant is screaming, a nurturing mother soothes him to lower his state of alarm. When the baby is depressed, an attuned mother raises his state to a more elevated mood. She does this naturally, without thinking about it. This helps the infant learn autoregulation of his own mood swings.

If the mother is emotionally unavailable, it is devastating. The psychological unavailability of the mother renders her infant emotionally, socially, and cognitively vulnerable. Because the child spends so much time trying to engage his mother, unavailability actually does more harm to the newborn than separation. Depressed mothers have difficulty responding to their babies, who either risk hurting themselves by becoming more violent, or completely withdraw to get attention.

The mother's mood is contagious. Infants begin to reflect it by the age of three months. When infants of stressed mothers were paired with nonstressed adults, their depressed style persisted. The behavior already had a permanent biological effect that was reflected by the differences in brain wave activity in the frontal lobe of the brain. Remember, such brain mapping occurs early and has lasting effects on later school performance and social interactions.

The infants of depressed mothers also had high salivary cortisol levels, which is an indication of stress reaction. One therapy for this is infant massage, which was developed by Dr. Fields. She did a well-controlled study on infants of depressed mothers and was able to demonstrate a change in their interaction and also a decrease in salivary cortisol levels in both mother and baby.

These well-done studies describing the importance of the maternal-infant interactions on the emotional development and later life behaviors can be extrapolated to the prenatal period. All the brain structures that control our emotions are well developed in utero. We neonatologists see the effects of pain, stress, and neglect on the premature infant's behavior. More importantly, we now know how to rebuild their disorganized brains by controlling the environmental stimulation they receive.

You, dear reader, cannot witness the devastation of stress on your unborn baby's behavior that I observe daily. But you have a great opportunity to begin nurturing the emotional development of your unborn child by taking fetal love breaks to flood your unborn child with your chemical fetal love messages.

Your love work is more effective before birth than after your child is born because your brain chemically communicates with him directly. After birth your parenting goal is to wash your child's brain with the same positive neuropeptides, but you can only do this indirectly, by communicating your love with your words and actions. I try to do the same in the intensive care nursery, so I know firsthand how difficult this is. Start now to use fetal love breaks to send your fetal love messages. They will alter his brain architecture and behavior for the rest of his life.

The Evolution of Our Emotions

A baby who is thought by many to be an unpretentious naked beginning of human development actually embodies the essentials for our continuing evolution. Our successful evolutionary strategy is the long immaturity period of infancy when we are excellent learners and are nurtured by adults who are eager to teach. Our ability to learn as babies and to teach as adults is the greatest advantage we have in evolutionary competition. Our most important and central instinct is the drive to learn.

A major educational advantage we have over other species on earth is the communication system we have to teach our young. The mammalian fetus is in a unique position of direct communication with its mother via the placenta, which allows the maternal systems to regulate the fetal physiology and development. This is done by the special production and then transfer of bioactive substances of many kinds that are important to fetal development and behavior. They also have long-term postnatal effects on health and behavior.

The impact of this prenatal communications system is greater on emotional tone than on cognitive abilities, because the emotional responses originate in the older parts of the brain structures that are relatively more mature at an earlier stage of fetal development. In this way our unborn child inherits the wisdom of our lives and is able to profit from it by preparing for the emotional content of the birth environment.

Why Do We Have Emotions?

So here you thought you only had to take care of your fetus's physical environment and now I tell you that emotions are possibly even more important. What next?

Have you ever wondered why we have emotions? Did evolutionary forces create them for us to enjoy or do they serve a purpose? Not all of them are enjoyable. So why do we have negative emotions? What good is it for us to feel angry, depressed, or stressed?

The short answer is that our emotions create our wisdom. They help us develop into individuals who can do wondrous acts. They give us the drive to achieve. They warn us of dangers. They help us understand other people. They enhance our memory. And, most important, they help us nurture our children—particularly the unborn child.

Like our spoken language, emotions helped us achieve our superior position in the animal kingdom. They are the language of our body's wisdom. Our emotions help us make the right decision by forcing us to contemplate our actions rather than merely to react to stimuli. Our emotions call us to rise above the instinctual behavior of lesser animals to develop our morality, which separates us from the rest of the animal kingdom. Albert Einstein stated it well: "Only morality in our actions can give beauty and dignity to our lives." Our emotions are carried by the neuropeptide molecules that cross the placenta to pass your wisdom to your unborn child. This biochemical mechanism for our emotions has been preserved through evolutionary history, which gave our ancestors a biological advantage for survival.

Emotions help us process information. For example, you and your infant see the same object, but because you are two different observers coming from two different experiences, you will see the same object—say, a red rubber ball—differently. The observer's frame of reference, based on different experiences and different emotional reactions, will set what each call their "reality."

This is similar to the prayer effect described in part 2. Prayer's action is not limited by time or space. It transcends them in ways difficult to understand. The reverse also happens in our bodies. A thought that is part of the nonphysical world can make a physical change in our bodies. We can blush when we have an embarrassing thought. The thought is a nonphysical entity that changes our body's physical bio-chemistry.

Have you ever walked into a room and felt an emotion emerge that you knew came from the people within it? It often happens to me when I am anticipating meeting loved ones or joining a party that I know will be fun and exciting. Scientists call this "emotional reso-nance"—basically feeling other people's emotions by a mechanism not yet fully understood.

Is it possible that our receptivity to this resonance has to do with the vibration of the receptor site in the neuropeptide system? I believe so. I also think this is the way prayer works. When we pray with faith and expectation, we set the tone of our receptor vibrations, which affects the response of the neuropeptides in our bodies.

Humans of all races and cultures use the same facial muscle for expressing emotions, and each of us can read facial expressions regard-less of language or cultural background. Charles Darwin noted in his book *Expression of Emotions in Man and Animals* that a wolf baring fangs uses the same facial muscles we do when we get angry. He con-cluded that emotions were used over and over during evolution, and therefore must have survival benefits.[4]

About a hundred years later, Candace Pert, Ph.D., discovered the neuropeptide system that is the biochemical mechanism for emotions throughout the animal kingdom, which confirmed Darwin's theory. All vertebrates, from the ugly and primitive hagfish to amphibians, reptiles, primates, and finally us humans, all share the same biochemi-cal system to express emotions.[5]

Most people think emotions to be uniquely human, but that is not correct as eloquently described by psychiatrist Dr. Jeffrey Moussaieff in his book *When Elephants Weep: The Emotional Lives of Animals*. Most pet owners will tell you with conviction that their pets have emotions.[6] So if all animals have the biochemical system to express emotions, why are we humans so superior? Our superiority comes from our ability to modulate our emotions. We use our brain's frontal lobe to further eval-uate what we are feeling and contemplate what if any action is needed. This refinement is based on our concepts (our wisdom) about our universe, which we collect through experience, the use of language, and, yes, prenatally from our mothers.

The midbrain's limbic system—the central hub of the neuroendocrine system and the seat of our emotions—and the brain's frontal lobes—the central hub for conscious decisions—are filled with neuropeptides and neuropeptide receptors. When we become emotionally excited, the limbic system becomes metabolically active and "lights up" on PET scans. When we think about what emotions we are feeling, their consequences, and what actions to take, the frontal lobes light up on PET scans. This interaction and coordination between the limbic system and the brain's frontal lobes allow us to ponder the consequences of our emotions, giving us humans an advantage over other primate species.

Our frontal lobes develop connections with the limbic system during the later part of gestation and during the first two years after birth. They finish their development when we are twenty years old. If the connections between the frontal lobes and the limbic system are not well developed by age two, many children become impulsively violent, and their frontal lobes don't "light up" the way they do in emotionally nurtured children. Basically, these unfortunate children are acting like they don't have the advantage of their frontal lobes.[7]

What Is Emotional Health?

For many, the concept of a healthy lifestyle is low-fat eating and daily exercise. Mind-body scientists think it involves more. They have clinical evidence to show that health involves the mind and spirit as well as the body. They claim that traditional medicine ignores the emotional and spiritual aspects of health and illness.

I agree with them and that is why I have included sections in this book on spirituality, prayer, and the healthy expression of our emotions. All these help control our thoughts and self-talk, which in turn greatly affect the neuroendocrine system in our bodies. We need to have the free expression of all emotions, including the so-called negative ones such as anger, grief, and fear. These emotions are not negative in themselves. They are important and serve us well. Anger helps defend our boundaries, grief helps us deal with losses, and fear protects us from danger. Like any other asset, they must be properly managed.

Illnesses occur when we deny our feelings and block neurotransmitter flow. Then the situation becomes toxic. This is why as a pregnant woman, you must learn to express your emotions freely and safely in relationships. The goal on the molecular level is to keep your neuropeptides moving and the feedback system working so your body returns to its tranquil state of health after an emotional experience. This is why it is important to feel safe in expressing your emotions to your life partner.

We are human "beings," not human "doings." Most of us spend too much time rushing about doing things, a common reaction to stress. We need to settle and quiet our minds and bodies in order to experience our feelings fully, be okay with them, and know that it is safe. Don't deny emotions but truly experience them. Fill your senses with them. This helps the feedback loops decrease the neuroendocrine system reaction; our emotions dissipate, their associated neurotransmitters are metabolized, and our cellular metabolism returns to its resting state. By expressing emotions you keep the feedback system functioning and the biochemical state of your cells continually updated and balanced—which is healthy for you, your family, and your unborn child.

We've covered a lot of ground so far in how your neuropeptides have a huge effect on your fetus both intellectually and emotionally. And there's still much more to go! Hang in there and keep reading and learning as we explore the powerful effect of the neuroendocrine system.

7

Emotional Communication with the Unborn Child

A belief which does not spring from conviction in the emotions is no belief at all.

—*Evelyn Scott Escapade*

Stress is a word with negative connotations. Some people physically react just hearing it. I've already shown you lots of ways stress can powerfully affect your fetus and continue to govern her development both intellectually and emotionally throughout life.

Certainly the world can be a stressful place to live, especially when you're pregnant. The good news, however, is that a great deal of stress is manageable, if not completely avoidable, depending on your actions and reactions. The remaining sections of this book are devoted to helping you find and practice the most beneficial ways to keep you and your developing fetus, as well as your supportive friends and family, less stressed.

But remember those neuropeptides I referred to a while ago? They're back! Actually, they never go away, and unfortunately, I have to start with stress neuropeptides. I would much rather write about positive neuropeptides, but medical science does not spend much time or money studying health. I do not present this information to scare you but rather to inform and empower you. At the end of this rather distressing section I promise you lots of valuable tips and techniques to ensure your unborn child's emotional health.

The Pharmacy in Our Head

Our brain is much more than a supercomputer of nerves acting like wires that carry impulses from one part of our body to another. Our brain is also a collection of glands that secrete chemicals called neuropeptides that affect many of our organs, especially the nervous system. This network of glands and the chemicals they secrete are called the neuroendocrine system.

The neuroendocrine system filters the information received by our nervous system by modifying the transmission of nerve impulses across the tiny gaps between our nerve cells. These junctions between nerve cells are called synapses. Each neuropeptide will affect in specific ways the nerve impulse as it crosses the synapse. One facilitates its passage, another diminishes it, a third completely blocks it. The larger the number of synapses along the path of the nerve impulse, the more influence the neuroendocrine system has on the bias and prioritization of the impulse's effect on the part of the brain it is racing toward.[1]

This neuropeptide filtering process helps us manage all the stimulation that bombards our nervous system. Otherwise we could not survive and prosper. Which neuropeptide is present when the nerve impulse arrives at the synapse impacts what we perceive and how we react to the stimulus. In this way our neuroendocrine system interprets our environment, which gives us wisdom. It coordinates our nervous, intestinal, endocrine, and immune systems, which all work together to help us be more competent in our world. The neuropeptides are best thought of as messenger molecules used to communicate among these important organs. The same neuropeptides are also called "molecules of emotion" because they create our emotions by affecting many of our organs that play a part in our emotional responses. When you get "that loving feeling" your "loving" neuropeptides are hard at work on the cell walls in a select group of your organs.

Neuropeptides cross the placenta to send messages to your unborn child. Once across the placenta they affect the transmission of nerve impulses in your unborn baby's nervous system and his other organs, just as they do yours. In this way your unborn child shares your emotional state. These neuropeptides also change the architecture of your unborn child's brain by altering the size, number, and connectivity of his nerve cells. In this way you pass the wisdom of your life experiences on to your unborn child. Your brain prepares the brain of your unborn child to perceive and react to his birth environment like you respond to your day-to-day situations.

Do not fret about the small temporary emotional stresses in your life, because the fetus's placenta protects him from temporary bursts of stress neuropeptides. Unfortunately, the placental barrier breaks down when there is chronic stress or fear in the mother's life. Once this happens the stress neuropeptides cross the placenta to alter the architecture of the child's developing brain.

If you do not know how to manage stress to change the neuropeptide mix in your body from that of stress and fear to one of love and peace, your neuropeptides will program your unborn infant's brain to expect stress and react fearfully to his birth environment. This is why the spiritual and psychological aspects of your pregnancy quest are so important. You have learned to use your neuropeptide system to send fetal love messages during fetal love breaks. In part 2 of this book you will learn how to build spiritual optimism and use prayer to control fear.

How Your Life Stress May Affect Your Unborn Child

We are all aware of the critical milestones in the neurodevelopment of our children—like walking at one year after birth. To begin to walk the infant needs to achieve several earlier milestones before successfully taking his first step. If any of these are not met, the likelihood of the child's walking diminishes.

In perinatal medicine we know that the developing fetus also passes through many development milestones before birth. Until the recent development in cellular biology, brain science, and medical imaging, brain scientists were under the misconception that this biological unfolding of our mental abilities was determined by the gene set we inherited from our parents. Now you have learned that this is only partly true and in some situations the environment of the developing fetus or child is more important to his long-term health than the genes he was dealt at conception. This is particularly true in emotional and intellectual development.

Our stress response is an important part of our emotional development. The problem is that its biology is rooted in the past and it does not adapt to the rapid changes occurring in our modern-day world. The stress response was appropriate when we resorted to physical activity in the face of danger. The mobilization of body fuels and the increase in blood pressure and heart rate prepare us for physical action. Now, because of our modern inactive way of life, the glucose, fatty acid, and neuropeptide surge in our bloodstream is not dissipated appropriately. Chronic stress changes our biochemistry, our brain architecture, and switches on dormant genes that leave memory traces in the brain.

Once our biochemistry, genes, and brains are set for stress, we react the same way to lesser stressors and the same memory traces are reinforced. Finally, after repeated reinforcements, the brain's memory traces take on a life of their own, which may permanently change the child's behavior and/or perception of his environment. Over our evolutionary history these changes in the infant's brain biology were beneficial, as in, say, a jungle environment. But in modern times this is not so, and the unfortunate child is birthed with maladaptive behavior patterns. He will aggressively react to stimuli that you and I would consider nonthreatening. (Does any of this start to sound increasingly important as we hear about more and more drugging of hyperactive children, or kids killing other kids with deadly weapons?)

The question often asked by my patients is: How much stress for how long causes these brain changes to my unborn child? The human data to answer this important question are sketchy. Women with high stress during pregnancies tend to birth hyperactive and developmentally delayed babies. The animal data on this issue are much more complete and quite convincing.

I tell patients that the stress is not as important as how they react to it. One mother can live in an environment and not show a stress response, while another mother will have a major stress reaction to the same situation. You will learn how to manage stress, even better than you already do. Do not worry about short episodes of stress, but be sure you reduce your neuropeptide surge using the techniques described in parts 2 and 3 of this book.

How Stress Affects Your Unborn Child

The animal research that supports the concepts about the adverse effects of maternal stress on pregnancy outcome is more prevalent and convincing in animals than in humans, because it is easier to research animals than humans.

Of course, we need to be careful when drawing conclusions from animal behavior research and applying them to human behavior. As I have described, the brains and placentas among species may differ. I try to point out these differences when they are known.

In spite of their limitations, the animal data are consistent in showing the adverse effects of stress on pregnancy outcome, particularly with the higher incidence of preterm births and low birth weights. The human data are less consistent for several reasons. First, we don't have good tools to measure and quantify stress. Most of the studies did not use physiologic markers to measure stress but rather psychological tools, which are imprecise and not easily quantified. The other variables in the human data are our ability to ameliorate the adverse effects of stress with many of the tools described later in this book such as meditation, positive self-talk, managing fear, and elevating self-esteem. Another confounding variable in the studies on humans is that most stressed humans have other behaviors, such as smoking or alcohol and drug use, that will also adversely affect pregnancy outcome. These risky behaviors may be caused by stress, which places it in the role of being an indirect cause of poor pregnancy outcome.

The Animal Data

All of the research presented is in primates and rats, because the rat and primate placentas metabolize cortisol, a stress neuropeptide, like the human placenta and can greatly affect these transgenerational studies of stress. I wish we had more data on the positive effects of the neuroendocrine system, but they are not available for the reasons stated previously. The message from these animal studies is that prenatal stress can permanently alter the newborn's stress response, but proper mothering immediately after birth can ameliorate this adverse condition in the brain and neuroendocrine system.

Rat Data

Young rats who were exposed prenatally to their mothers' stress neuropeptides had exaggerated responses to stress after birth when compared to the pups whose mothers were not stressed. The prenatally stressed pups had changes in the hippocampus area of their brains and to their neuroendocrine systems. Their stress responses remained exaggerated long after the prenatal exposure. When the brains of the prenatally stressed pups were studied, the researchers found them to be less sensitive to their own stress neuropeptides, and their neuroendocrine systems were in high gear, producing an abundance of stress neuropeptides that kept their metabolisms and sensory organs in a hyperacute state. A stimulus that normally would not cause a stress response did so in these rat pups exposed to prenatal stress. These rat pups also developed hypertension later in life.[2]

Other rat studies show that prenatally stressed pups who received from their mothers an increased amount of licking and grooming (rat "motherese") had their neuroendocrine systems' set point for stress lowered, and they had a normal stress response later in life. This shows that the prenatal programming can be altered by postnatal maternal behavior. The more licking by the pups' mothers, the lower the set point.

The message is that stress may change your unborn child's brain and neuroendocrine system, but after his birth you can alter his stress response. This window of opportunity lasts for about two years in the human infant. After that time it becomes much harder to change a child's temperament.

Monkey Data

The research on primates indicates that prenatal stress is a factor that predisposes young monkeys to aggressive behaviors. After birth, the monkeys not properly parented had brains that were wired differently from ones that had good parenting. They had the same kind of brain damage as seen in the rat pups exposed to severe stress.

Dr. Clark, a brain research scientist, removed pregnant rhesus monkeys from their cages and exposed them to unpredictable loud bursts of noise three times a day. This produced a stress reaction in the mother monkeys and increased the blood levels of stress neuropeptides in their fetuses. After birth, the prenatally stressed monkeys showed extreme stress and exaggerated emotional reactions when compared to a control group of young monkeys whose mothers were not stressed by the loud noise.[3]

The researchers conclude that the mother's stress hormones had a negative effect on the developing fetal brain, which later affected the monkey's reaction to stress. The prenatally stressed monkeys had less adaptive social behaviors and higher risk for aggressive behaviors that led four of the prenatally stressed monkeys to attempt or actually kill their cage mates. This violent behavior was not predicted by the researchers and they stopped the research for ethical reasons.

In another study, at the University of Wisconsin, brain scientists found that the earlier the stress in gestation, the more intense the symptoms. The prenatally stressed monkeys, as in Dr. Clark's experiment, showed increased stress reactions after birth. They also had poor social skills and tended to be disruptive in the monkey colony and to their cage mates.

Human Data

A mother's stress neuropeptides may be transferred to her fetus if their concentration overloads the placenta's ability to metabolize them. Mary Schneider at the University of Wisconsin found that stress neuropeptide levels increased in a fetus if his mother was exposed to significant stresses during pregnancy. When a pregnant mother becomes stressed, the fact that she is stressed is not as important as how quickly and how well she is able to manage the stress and reduce the stress neuropeptides in her body.

When she is able to recognize she is stressed and uses techniques to reduce the neuropeptide surge and keep the neuroendocrine system in balance, she bathes her unborn infant's brain with comforting neuropeptides. This teaches both brains that stress is okay, because there is recovery from it. The main problems come from chronic stress that is never relieved.

Dr. Heidi Als at Harvard Medical School has studied the long-term effects of stress in premature infants. Her carefully controlled, multicenter research demonstrated that premature infants who did not receive the nurturing techniques of reducing their stress reaction to their neonatal intensive care environment had poor school performance and slow neurodevelopment. The premature infants who were cared for by nurses who looked for and relieved the infants' stress reactions had much better neurological outcomes. They not only did better in school but also on the psychological tests administered. Their emotional responses to other children were better modulated. They were less impulsive, had better-organized motor behaviors, and were better able to concentrate and complete academic tasks.[4]

Emotional Retardation

There is something fundamental about our relationships with our parents that reverberates through the rest of our lives. Parenting has a major impact on our physical and emotional survival. Caregivers send subtle messages of emotional comfort to the developing brain that sets an emotional balance point. A mother's ability to read cues from her baby and respond to them modulates the stress neuropeptides effects on the key emotional centers of the infant's brain. Her sensitivity and responsiveness sculpt her child's brain circuits.

An infant left to cry endlessly or whose cry is met with a slap has a brain reaction that differs from that of the child who is properly nurtured. These reactions become the biological foundation of the child's emotional balance. The brain architecture in the prefrontal cortex can be altered by parental neglect or destroyed by chronic stress. In both situations the child develops emotional retardation in the form of inability to trust others or to express empathy. They have learned their universe is not safe!

The prenatal and early parent-infant interaction creates in the baby a neuropsychological state similar to his mother's. T. Berry Brazelton has shown this in his videotaping of generations of mothers. The children who were mothered well tended to mother better than the children who were not. In fact, the young mothers tended to mirror the posture and the techniques used on them by their mothers even though they had never seen videos of themselves being mothered. The similarity in behaviors was uncanny. How the newborn remembers and subconsciously duplicates the same techniques was remarkable. The posture and handling were so similar that researchers think the memory was somatic.[5]

Like the unfortunate situation of mental retardation, the degree of injury from stress depends on the circumstances and the age of the child. The younger the child, the more likely the stress will affect the lower brain centers, which makes the responses later in the infant's development stronger and more primitive. The prenatal stress response in the brain stem and midbrain alters the later development of the brain cortex, which perpetuates the child's aggressive behaviors.

Our ability to think before we respond to perceived danger depends on the ratio between the excitatory activity of the midbrain and the moderating effects of its cortex—particularly the frontal lobes of the cortex. Chronic stress increases the excitatory activity of the primitive brain and decreases the regulating activity of the frontal lobes. Both of these stress effects lead to aggressive impulsive behaviors.

A child can have so much stress in his life that his midbrain is constantly in a hyperalert state of vigilance, always looking from a fearful frame at his environment, and continually sending alarm signals to the rest of his body. This constant stimulation pulls neural circuits away from other functions like memory to strengthen the ones that help him respond to his perceived perils. If this goes too far his brain will surrender and crumble. The child shuts down emotionally. He gives up.

I see this in the extremely sick premature infants who are stressed in our nursery. We call it "falling apart" and usually it takes only several days. For years we thought this was a natural progression of their illnesses, but now we know this is a response to the extreme stress of being born too early.

If infants remain in the "falling apart" period too long, they never reorganize their brain and have lifelong effects from the experience as described by Dr. Heidi Als. Modern neonatology is excellent in saving premature infants and we have come a long way in preventing severe neurological handicaps, but the majority of our extremely premature infants who graduate from their intensive care experience are having problems with hyperactivity, easy distractibility, and interpersonal relations—all directly related to their stress experience right after birth. These kids have difficulty learning empathy and emotional attachment to others. They have trouble controlling and balancing feelings in interpersonal relations.

The same can happen to the developing brain of an unborn child. It is true that a child in utero is better protected from stress than a premature infant. You have read about the effects of chronic stress on the brain of an unborn child. But you can not experience what I must while caring for my tiny stressed patients. If you could watch these same dramatic changes in your unborn child's behavior, you would better understand the compelling force that drives me to toil late into the night writing this book. My patients' distress would call you to do whatever you could to prevent the same from happening to your unborn child.

We have all read about parents heroically saving their children. The danger and their frantic children call these parents to action. My prayer is that these words become the distress cry from your unborn child that calls you to make your body a peaceful womb for your developing child.

Birth Memories

Dr. David Chamberlain, a psychologist, used hypnosis to regress patients back to their births, and they report amazingly accurate memories that revealed lucid thoughts and feelings at the time of birth.[6]

An important new body of evidence for the reality of birth memories is the spontaneous recounting of them by toddlers from two to three years old. A good time to try this with your children is when they are ready for bed or during a playful bath. The obvious question is, are they real and accurate? Many parents have been astounded at how accurate they are.

To answer this question, Dr. Chamberlain studied ten pairs of mothers and their grown children. Both mother and child had to meet three criteria to be studied. Both had to be capable of hyperamnesia, which is the ability to recall vivid and complete memories under hypnosis. The mothers had to assure him that nothing about the birth was told to the children, and the child had no conscious birth memory. The children ranged from age nine to twenty-three, and the mothers from thirty-two to forty-six years old.

The mother's memory was assumed to be reliable and the child's was compared for accuracy. The reports validated each other in many details with similar memories outnumbering the contradictions. Four of the ten pairs had no contradictions in their memories. Five had only one contradiction, and one pair had four contradictions. Dr. Chamberlain concludes, "Taking the reports as a whole, they appear to be coherent, overlapping, and generally accurate."

Dr. Chamberlain's work shows that babies can remember events and are capable of receiving and giving messages by using and reading body language. Many birth memories are like near-death experiences. Some children were able to display a wisdom that could not be explained. They knew facts, explained possibilities, and recited the thoughts and feelings of the people involved in the delivery. His studies suggest that babies are conscious at birth and have intelligence as well as wisdom. From my personal experience in interviewing families who have asked their toddlers about their births, I believe that infants do remember their births.

To accept this work as true, we must understand that our communication goes well beyond the words we use. Throughout the animal kingdom communication is done by scents, body postures, facial expressions, and eye contact. All of this is available to the newborn. I often feel I communicate with my patients. I have given them thoughts of love, sympathy, understanding, and watched closely as their faces changed and their bodies relaxed. Newborns, you will soon learn, can communicate their desires with their eyes, faces, body posture, hands and feet.

I conclude from these data that newborns have an identity, they act mindfully, and they can communicate in sophisticated ways. These qualities are fragile and can easily be lost, but babies are far more capable than we used to believe.

The brains of children from stressful pregnancies are different. So are their lives. They have trouble concentrating on tasks such as schoolwork. Many of them seek constant stimulation like loud music or drugs. It is the only way they can quiet their brains. These are the very kids who get in trouble because they misinterpret the social cues from other children in the schoolyard. They always think they are being attacked or persecuted and usually get in trouble, which only reinforces the stress and surge of neuropeptides that is driving the brain to hyper-alert states. Most of us, who are stressed at one time or another, recover and our cortisol and noradrenaline levels in our bloodstream and brain go down, but these children living in chronic stress have high levels of cortisol and adrenaline for long periods of time.

Severe depression during pregnancy leads to increased cortisol levels that can adversely affect the development of the infant's emotional networks. Clinical studies of infants delivered by depressed mothers show they have lower electrical activity in brain areas that regulate joy, happiness, and curiosity. The longer their mothers remain depressed, the higher the likelihood of the child's becoming depressed. A follow-up study of children at the University of Washington showed that at three years of age these children were more likely to be withdrawn, disobedient, aggressive, and to have behavior problems such as crying and not sleeping. These children have higher levels of stress neuropeptides.

After birth the emotionally unavailable mother is more devastating to the newborn than one who is absent, because the child spends so much time trying to engage his depressed mother. Babies experiment until they find the behavior that communicates best with their parents, and parents quickly learn how to read and respond to these infant cues. A depressed mother is not able to respond to her infant's behavior cues. The infant's feelings may not be recognized and eventually he will shut down emotionally.

Infants do this slowly. They begin by showing less motor activity and less eye contact and finally totally withdraw. Some mothers respond erratically to their infants, which makes the situation worse. Giving pregnant women and mothers with young infants their emotional needs and sense of security is important. It reduces their stress hormones and alters their baby's developing brain's chemistry and architecture.

The negative effects of prolonged stress on infants can be reduced by placing the infant with nonstressed or cheerful caregivers for long periods of time. A better option is to get the depressed mother into therapy and on medication. I have seen dramatic effects on infant behavior when a depressed or chronically anxious mother is successfully treated. She becomes emotionally available and the infant begins to thrive on his mother's emotional feedback.

Dr. Allen Schore at UCLA School of Medicine thinks the frontal lobe of the cortex is the key area in both infant attachment and emotional regulation. It receives both external sensory stimulation and visceral information from the body's internal environment. It connects the facial expression of mother with what the infant is feeling at the time. If it is intense pleasure, one set of nerve fibers are enhanced; if it is intense pain or fear, a different set is cultivated.[7]

The fibers in this area are especially sensitive to the emotional expressions of the human face, and are strongly connected to centers in the midbrain where strong emotions are generated. The frontal cortex develops at the time infant-mother attachment is evolving. Its structure is dependent on the quality of their relationship and sets the core for later development of emotional relationships. An early positive emotional experience shapes the infant's lifelong ability to modulate and nurture all relationships. The underactivity of the frontal cortex and overactivity of the midbrain can be seen on the PET scans of impulsive killers.

Dr. Adrian Raine did PET scans of twenty-two convicted California murders and found that the prefrontal lobes of these criminal brains were either overaroused in those who committed hot-blooded, impulsive murders or underaroused in the calculating perpetrators of cold-blooded murders. These findings coincided with a particular neuropeptide mix. High noradrenaline and low serotonin levels were present in the hot-blooded criminals, while the cold-blooded premeditated murderers, who lacked remorse and emotion, had low noradrenaline and serotonin levels. A person with a normal serotonin level will stop and think about what he or she is doing.[8] Children with normal noradrenaline levels will remain calm in stressful situations if they are with a parent with whom they feel safe. If the child is in an environment in which he does not feel safe, the noradrenaline level goes up, as does the hyperactive aggressive behavior.

Part II

The Peaceful Womb

$\mathcal{C}$hoosing the Road to Birthing a Healthy Baby

Give all to love; obey thy heart.

—*Ralph Waldo Emerson*

"Health care" is fulfilling your potential, the optimal development of your physical, psychological, and spiritual talents. Providers of health care are well educated and highly trained. Our formal education about diseases and their treatment continues twelve to fifteen years beyond high school. But what health care consumers are learning—though unfortunately most of my colleagues have not—is that treating diseases is a different enterprise from providing "health care." Physicians tend to deal with "disease care," which is the application of medical science and technology to treat sick patients.

If you have a disease, going to a physician is an excellent decision, but health is much more than just the absence of disease. I am a physician committed to "health care," and this book is your self-directed guide to achieving optimal health for you and your unborn child during pregnancy.

Most of us don't appreciate the importance of our health. We take it for granted and do very little to improve it until it is threatened or we lose it. Then it becomes paramount, but unfortunately, the suggested prevention initiatives are often not as effective after disease develops.

This section presents scientific information about prayer, controlling fears, and self-talk. These are the keys to making good decisions, changing behaviors, and effectively communicating with your life partner, your medical team, and your unborn child. In part 3 I describe a daily routine to help you physically, mentally, and spiritually prepare for your pregnancy and labor. By following the prescribed routines, you cannot help but improve your birthing experience as well as the health and happiness of your unborn child. The work of making these changes is truly fetal love work, which requires unconditional love.

I want to help you explore more than the physical aspects of your pregnancy. Let's explore your thoughts, fears, and values that are important in clinical decision making. If you are not interested in making decisions, changing unwanted behaviors, or using your natural abilities to take charge of birthing a healthy full-term infant, but instead are relying solely on your medical team for your health care, please reexamine your decisions. We health care providers can't control the outcome of your pregnancy. Only you and your loved ones can do that.

You probably have many thoughts and questions, both simple and complex. Write them in your pregnancy notebook now. Questions may come to you at times when you have no one to turn to for an answer. Make a list of them to discuss when you visit your health care provider. Questions I am often asked are: Did I do something wrong, or, What if I do something that may hurt my baby? And, Will I be able to manage the pain of labor? Will my partner help me? Will my parents and friends support me?

And the questions continue. As a father four times, I had them. My wife had them. My patients' families have them. I have learned much in our search for the answers. Here are our collective thoughts about the major issues we all face when pregnant.

The Basic Question

What am I? Men and women have contemplated this fundamental question since the beginning of human thought. It has been discussed in the world's great literature among the distinguished thinkers of ancient cultures and contemporary philosophers from Aristotle to Einstein. It is an important question for each of us to contemplate.

The question What am I? is much different from the question

Who am I? The latter is easy to answer because it describes what we do, who we are related to, the color of our skin, our nationality, among other factors. However, none of these descriptions tells us what we are.

The What am I? query goes to the center of our being, our essence, our soul. The great philosophers of the world, both secular and religious, have several different answers, but I think one of the best answers was given by Ralph Waldo Emerson when he stated, "Man is a piece of the universe made alive."

Pregnancy is a unique state, one that offers opportunities as well as challenges. It is common for first-time pregnant parents to look at their lives differently, and to examine fundamental questions such as this one. They sense an awakening of new life, of importance, of responsibility, and of the perplexity of the magnificent changes occurring in and around them.

The concept of self or What am I? is the core of our being. The question triggers many of our responses to common life situations like relating to loved ones, selecting a spouse, deciding to have sex, or becoming pregnant. Our answer determines how we respond to others and to our environment. It shapes our happiness, our successes, our failures—basically, the future of our lives, and to a great extent, the outcome of a pregnancy. The question What am I? is so vital to our lives that we all need to answer it; and the younger we are when we grapple with it, the more successful we are likely to be in every aspect of our lives, from personal relationships to financial rewards. So let's get to work answering it.

Think back to Emerson's words: "I am the universe made alive." Let them sink into your mind. Repeat them silently as you see them in your mind's eye. Open your perspective to the possibilities of what the statement might mean. After relaxing and thinking about them, record your thoughts. Let them flow onto the paper, so you can come back to ponder them later.

Is the Universe a Friendly Place to Live?

Albert Einstein was once asked by a newspaper reporter what the most important question was for man to answer. To the surprise of everyone at the press conference, Einstein quickly answered, "The most important question for man to answer is whether the universe is a friendly place."

What do you think? Is your universe friendly?

When I think of the universe, my mind's eye sees the night sky with galaxies sprinkled in indescribable vastness filled with unfathomable black holes and quasars. At first, I had problems with the concept that I am the universe made alive, but after further thought, the concept gives me comfort and assurance that I am okay, and the universe is a friendly place to live.

The statement "I am the universe made alive" lifts you to a pinnacle of importance that may be hard to understand or believe. Can it be that you are important to the universe? Can your thoughts and actions affect it? To answer these questions, let's explore some facts about each of us and the earth.

Among modern astrophysicists there is a developing consensus that the universe, during its thirteen-billion-year evolution, was aligned toward the goal of creating human life.[1] Any minor deviations in many of the laws of physics such as the gravitational constant, electromagnetism, or in the precise ratios of the weights of subatomic particles, which all originated in its beginning, would have created an unrecognizable universe without stars, atoms, or life.[2]

The strange and extremely improbable coincidences in the values at the vast astrophysical level as well as at the incredibly minuscule atomic level have led astronomers and physicists to the same conclusion: "The universe has to know in advance what it is going to be before it knows how to start itself." They further conclude, "The most basic explanation of the universe is that it seems to be a process orchestrated to achieve the end or goal of creating human beings.[3]

The above consensus about the universe's origin applies to you gestating a baby. They are both processes that originate with the intent of creating a human being. You, being pregnant, are the universe made alive!

Our planet is unique. There is no other known place in the universe that supports life. Even as our earth is distinct in the universe, so is each of us unique. No two people are alike, not even identical twins. We each have our own individual habits, likes, dislikes, beliefs, and fears. Each of us has unique talents and gifts possessed from birth that are singularly ours to use as we choose for the rest of our lives. But how we use them is important. Like a pebble dropped into a pool of water, the ripples of our thoughts and actions send out ever-expanding waves of influence to all things around us, seen and unseen, known and unknown.

No thought is without its effect on us, the people around us, and then the people around them. Like the pebble dropped into the pool of water, what each of us does has its ripple effect, ever expanding into our universe. We are important—each of us—to our unborn children, to our families and friends, to our neighborhoods, to this earth, and, yes, to the universe. Just as your developing fetus is created by you and will become your child at birth, we were created by and are all children of the universe. Emerson was writing in these terms when he stated "Man is the universe made alive."

How should we name this great power that birthed us and the universe? Author Vladimir Nabokov put these words into the mouth of Kinbote in his book *Pale Fire:* "I know . . . that the world could not have occurred fortuitously and that somehow Mind is involved as a main factor in the making of the universe. In trying to find the right name for that Universal Mind, or First Cause, or the Absolute, or Nature, I submit that the name of God has priority."[4]

My own personal belief is in this God as Creator. You may use the term universe, ultimate provider, higher power, or God, or whatever name you prefer. The important concept here is that there is a magnificent power that has created all that we see, know, and understand. How you view that power and your relationship to it is all-important to you, to this pregnancy, and to your unborn child.

This doesn't mean that we are equal with God, no more than one can say that a sea wave is the ocean; but as waves are to the ocean, we are to the universe. No two people are alike as no two waves are alike, and yet each is part of a larger more magnificent whole. The wave cannot be the ocean, it is only one part of it, and at the same time one with it. We individuals are not and cannot be God, but we are part of and can be one with God.

The Universal Composition of Matter

Let's switch from personal views to scientific study for a bit. All the universe is made up of the same basic atoms that we studied on the periodic table in high school chemistry class. The congregation of atoms amassed in us is no different than those assembled in the earth, planets, sun, and stars. These basic elements make up all matter throughout the universe.

A startling visual presentation of this concept is expressed in the popular book *Powers of Ten, About the Relative Size of Things in the Universe.*[5] It contains a series of spectacular photographs that start with a telescopic view of a distant galaxy in space. Each picture is reduced by one tenth in power until the picture comes to a view of Earth from satellite photographs, then aerial photographs, and finally to a scene in normal perspective of a young couple sitting on a blanket in a park.

The next series of photographs start magnifying the viewer's perspective by the power of ten. From the park scene, the views are of a close-up of the man's skin, then the cells of his skin, then the cellular structure, and finally into the smallest structures that an electron microscope can detect in the nucleus of a skin cell. At the two extremes of power in the pictorial essay an amazing fact becomes apparent: the far limits of the universe look similar to the tiniest, subatomic details of the cellular structure of our bodies.

Science is now teaching us that the human body, like all matter, is primarily made up of space filled with energy fields. The actual mass of our molecules is small in comparison to the space occupied by the energy fields around their atoms and subatomic particles. To put this in perspective, one scientist describes the nucleus of an atom as being like a golf ball in the center of the Houston Astrodome, with the nearest electron circling around it just above the stadium's roof. The rest of the space in our bodies is filled with energy fields that are frequently altered by the biochemical reactions we can control with the mental exercises you will learn.

These atoms flow back and forth between the living and nonliving segments of our earth. They are conserved and reused in very efficient and effective ways. Take the carbon atom as an example. It is fundamental to living organisms and to many nonliving structures. We exhale carbon atoms as carbon dioxide. In turn, plants assimilate our excreted carbon atoms into their fruits and vegetables, which we eat, digest, and use to build protein molecules in organs such as our muscles. Once the muscle uses the energy in the ingested plant sugar, the carbon atom is again excreted as carbon dioxide.

All living matter shares the same atoms in the same way. Your brain probably is using the same atoms that were once used by the great thinkers throughout history. We are interconnected with all that is alive, with our planet earth—and probably with the entire universe.

In a fundamental way we are like all other matter in the cosmos, truly children of the universe. All matter is primarily fields of energy that occupy relatively vast space between subatomic components. This is true from tiny atoms to the vast galaxies in the cosmos. But we are more than just pieces of universal matter. Each of us is a unique, vital cluster of elements filled with energy that is able to think, communicate, and birth. We are small pieces of the universe made alive; and yet, more than that, because we resemble our Creator more than any other part of the universe.

We are able to love, to procreate, and, yes, to hate and destroy. We have free will and can choose between good or evil. We have choices in how we react to the events in our lives, how we think, and how we use the energy in our minds and bodies. These choices affect the cells in our bodies and those of our loved ones, our families, and without question our unborn children. Nothing else in creation has that ability. We are important and, in many ways, we reflect our Creator.

Our Mind's Power of Choice

God has given us awesome power and responsibility that is not present anywhere else. Think of an angry ocean that can easily destroy beaches, towns, and humans. But the ocean also has the wonderful ability to support abundant life, in fact more plentifully than any other part of the universe. The ocean is the earth's greatest resource of life and needs respect and care from all of us.

Like the ocean, we also have the power to both create and destroy. The main difference is that we have the ability to choose how we use our power, whereas the ocean does not. It passively reacts to circumstances outside itself, like the wind, the gravitational forces of the moon and sun, and earthquakes. We have free will and complete control over our thoughts and attitudes, which, in turn, control our actions that ultimately control our life's circumstances.

We make simple choices daily. Am I going to be loving and happy, or am I going to be afraid and angry? Some of us may think events and people outside of ourselves determine our emotions, like love and anger, but in reality, we choose to be angry or loving regardless of the circumstances. Each time we choose, we express our power, which controls our actions, our lives, and how people react to us. Eventually, like the ripple effect, how we relate to the universe and, by the law of cause and effect, how it reacts to us, depend on our choices.

Victor Frankl, author of the outstanding book *Man's Search for Meaning*,[6] talks about the importance of our freedom to control our thoughts. He reports that in the Nazi concentration camps during World War II, living conditions were the worst the modern world had experienced, and yet there was a group of men who seemed to rise above the situation. They had an inner strength that protected them from the pestilence and diseases of the crowded, filthy camps of undernourished men. His cohort of fellow prisoners made conscious choices to create value out of the horrific circumstances surrounding their lives.

The Nazi guards stripped these prisoners of the freedoms that you and I enjoy, except the last freedom, the one that cannot be taken away from any of us—our personal thoughts about what is happening in our lives. In those horrible conditions, prisoners still had the choice of what attitude they embraced, as they endured each day filled with death and suffering. Not even the guards, nor the death stench surrounding them, could take away their spiritual optimism. They were able to say yes to their universe and to see value in their experiences, which helped them survive the pestilence, the torture, and the death chambers.

If Frankl and others could create something positive out of life in the Nazi death camps, then all of us have the ability to create value out of anything life hands us. It is a matter of remaining conscious that we have a choice. It is as simple as that. We may not control what happens to us in life, but we can choose how we react to it.

Birth as a Rite of Passage

Abraham H. Maslow states in his book *Motivation and Personality*[7] that we have a hierarchical system of biological drives that affects our behaviors. Once our basic needs, such as food and shelter, are satisfied, we will search for our need that is next in importance. This system of biological needs ultimately leads us to search for the personal and spiritual meanings of our lives.

This innate drive, expressed in all world cultures, is coded in the genetic material present in each of our cells. It is as much a part of us as the migration patterns of birds is to them. And although we each feel alone on these internal quests for meaning in our lives, we should remember that this force has been experienced by generation after generation of our ancestors. It is part of the collective consciousness we share with all mankind.

When the natural evolution of our biological drives is thwarted at a low level, we are left in the vague abyss of empty loneliness, due to our ignorance about the meaning of life. If the abyss is not eventually filled with love and understanding so that we may move upward along Maslow's hierarchy, depression may be the result.

Many adults searching for meaning in their lives come to the dismal question, Is this all there is to life? Nothing satisfies them. They are malcontent and search for worldly pleasures to fulfill their needs and appease their searching. But ultimately it's a futile attempt to fill the void, this abyss of loneliness. Some call this a "midlife crisis," and some call it "mental illness."

As a society, we seem to have little tolerance for people who are on this exploratory quest, which is unfortunate, because many of these people return to society with new purpose and direction, similar to the internal transition of the heroes or heroines in the quest analogy we looked at earlier. We need to change our perspectives toward those going through this growth process, a process that is accepted in most primitive societies as "rites of passage."

A rite of passage has three distinct stages. The first is the separation of the initiate from his or her previous place in the society. This usually involves a period of isolation or incarceration. Until recently we in our society have done this with pregnancy, or what we used to call "the period of confinement." We still use the term *expected date of confinement* or "EDC" in perinatal medicine.

The second stage of a rite of passage is the liminal phase, when the initiate is between the old stage of life and the higher, enlightened period of life. Older cultural traditions give important positive meaning to this natural maturational process. They view those in the liminal stage as we might view a developing fetus in the womb—readying themselves for a transition or rebirth into a new world of experience and understanding.

Pregnancy brings us to a point in our lives that some would call a rite of passage. Don't be surprised that you may feel alone and afraid during your pregnancy. It is important to recognize these feelings, to see them as part of a positive process of change, and then to take the appropriate steps to seek help from loved ones during the process.

Pain is part of this rite of passage, as it is in all important life transitions like birth and death. There's a painful period of darkness when the initiate, or neonate, has to let go of what is known to acquire higher understanding and a refurbished life. Your baby will soon leave the safety of your uterus and placenta (the utero-placental unit), which superbly performs many important biological functions such as respiration, temperature control, digestion, and excretion. He doesn't expend the energy you and I do on these and many other important bodily functions. He's on easy street in one of the universe's most pristine sustenance sources—the placenta, which prepares his nutrition in its most desirable biological form.

Soon he will emerge from this magnificent sanctuary with his own rite of passage textured with profound biological and psychological adjustments. As with most rites of passage, he will experience pain during his birth, but he is biologically equipped with an abundance of the neuropeptide endorphin, the natural opiate to dull the pain's intensity. These are the same brain opiates you can release during labor by using mental imagery and relaxation techniques. Fortunately, most who pass through these periods of transition arrive at the third stage of the rite of passage when they rejoin society in a new role, with a new perspective, and are endowed with a newly acquired importance. This is certainly the case for the fetus. Once he is born, he gains value and status that he did not have before birth. His birth confers a set of laws to protect him. He has completed a biological process and a societal rite of passage that give him added importance and status not enjoyed prior to birth.

In *The Power of Myth*, Joseph Campbell states, "The one thing that is constant in all myths of the world is that at the bottom of the abyss comes the voice of salvation."[8] At our darkest moments of despair comes the light of understanding. The same thought is expressed in the poem *The Prophet*, where Kahlil Gibran states, "Pain is the bitter pill of the inner physician that cracks the shell of our understanding."[9] How can a seed grow into a flower unless the seed swells and dies? Learning new ways to live and love is associated with crises and pain that force us to let go of old behaviors and beliefs in order to pass over a threshold to new understanding. This is the quest story's inner passage of growth that transcends all societies.

In Western society we seem to have lost our appreciation of darkness as a process for finding light, and yet that is exactly the psychological evolution commonly experienced by pregnant couples gestating and birthing their children. The word *pregnant* means having possibilities of development, resourcefulness, rich in significance, momentous. It is a significant period, rich in momentous possibilities for psychological and spiritual development. You must be willing to forgo old concepts to learn new ones. This can be painful, but like your unborn child you have the capacity to endure it. How can you make this pregnancy a significant life passage? As your trailblazer, I'd like to show you some ways to use your innate wisdom to do exactly that.

9

$\mathcal{F}$aith, Prayer, and Love

Prayer is the umbilical cord that allows you with your embryonic ideas, to draw nourishment from a source that you, like an unborn infant, can neither see nor fully know or comprehend, God our heavenly Father!
—*Dr. Robert Schuller*

Faith and prayer are pivotal to my belief that you can increase the safety of your pregnancy by taking more responsibility for its outcome. Thinking you are incapable of handling such responsibility will only work against you. You must have faith in your ability to do this.

True, a better understanding of what is going on with the pregnancy and how to manage the pain of labor will help you achieve your goal of birthing a healthy baby. But the critical breakthrough is to realize fully that you and your loved ones are more important to your pregnancy quest than are the medical team and hospital you select.

First trust the universe, and rely on a power greater than yourself and your medical team. It may seem paradoxical to surrender the outcome of your pregnancy to a greater power while at the same time being asked to take charge of its outcome. But this is not contradictory. You can't give away anything you don't possess, so you first must assume responsibility, before you can legitimately and faithfully entrust it to God.

This is an important step only you can take. Giving the medical establishment the responsibility for your pregnancy is not the same as your believing that you are capable of handling the situation. Only you can change unwanted behaviors that can adversely affect your baby. Only you can maintain a proper diet, recognize the early signs of premature labor, keep your prenatal appointments, and properly take prescribed medications. Only you can take fetal love breaks, manage your fears, build your self-esteem, practice mental imagery and relaxation, and finally be mentally tough enough to do the work necessary to deliver your infant. What a privilege to have such responsibility for gestating and birthing your child. Seize it and call on your higher power to give you the strength and wisdom to accomplish this important task of unconditional fetal love work.

Write these sentence stems on the top of a page in your journal and complete them with as many ideas as come to you.

To me, God is . . .

Prayer is useful when . . .

If you have trouble with these sentence stems and you cannot honestly answer Dr. Einstein's question about the universe's safety, then you may have doubts about your ability to meet the challenges of childbearing and -rearing. These daunting responsibilities can create fear and stress in your mind that may have devastating effects on your unborn child's developing brain. Using prayer to build spiritual optimism is the best way to assume these awesome responsibilities while creating a peaceful womb. When you are at peace, so is your unborn child.

Prayer with Faith Affects Medical Outcomes

Most people think prayer involves talking to some sort of authoritative, white, male, cosmic figure who prefers English. For most of my life I thought that prayer was basically a matter of faith. I grew up in the Episcopal Church, but I stopped attending while in college and medical school. It was not until ten years later, when I was in my fellowship in neonatal-perinatal medicine, that I returned to the church and found prayer to be meaningful.

During college and medical school I was influenced by many of my teachers who were committed to the pursuit of pure science, and had no tolerance for the mysteries of religion. They pursued the cause-

and-effect relationships in medicine that could be analyzed and statistically quantified in the laboratory. The discipline of the scientific method was important training for me. I needed to know how to evaluate the clinical literature so that I could make rational medical decisions based on scientific evidence. My job was to apply evidence-based medical theory to my patients, and there was no tolerance for the application of religion and spirituality.

But I found that, contrary to my training in scientific methods, there were incidences in my clinical practice when I was medically certain that a patient would die, only to have the baby survive. Typically, I would tell a family that there was nothing more medical science had to offer their child, and that I expected she would die. Some of these families asked if they could come into the nursery to be with their dying baby and to pray. To my amazement and that of my colleagues, some of these critically ill infants survived their illnesses. These unexplained survivals so impressed me, that I started asking families to sit by their child's bedside to console and nurture her while we continued to try to effect a medical cure.

The benefit of the family's prayers was consistent enough to pique my curiosity. I began to investigate the literature about the power of prayer. To my surprise, I learned that there are over 130 studies that statistically prove prayer's effect. Some of them are well-designed medical studies, which eliminate all other explanations for the patients' improvements.[1]

Understanding Prayer

Perhaps you have had some bad experiences with prayer, but I want to encourage you to try it again during your pregnancy. On the other hand, I am NOT advocating abandoning conventional medical wisdom and technology. I AM encouraging you to use prayer and meditation in addition to what is offered by modern medical science. This is becoming more commonplace as the spiritual movement continues in this country. The governmental medical insurance program in England, for example, already pays for the visit of a spiritual healer to hospitalized patients.

Some people have problems with prayer from a lack of understanding. Here are some of the common misconceptions I've seen.

Prayer without faith will not work. There is no question that faith is the power behind prayer and will help individuals achieve their goals when they firmly believe they have a relationship with God—a partnership, so to speak. There are several studies that document love and compassion as being more important than faith in achieving a measurable response to prayer. Most of these studies are done on bacteria and plants, living organisms that don't have the capacity of faith and cannot be affected by the knowledge that someone is praying for them.

In these studies, there was no advantage of one type of theology or method of praying over another. Groups of people from all different religions and beliefs were able to create the same changes in the test subjects. Interestingly, agnostics who expressed compassion and love for the seeds, plants, and bacteria were just as effective as those who had a firm belief in a deity or supreme being.

Prayer is wishful thinking. Many people have trouble asking for something during prayer because they think it is nothing more than wishful thinking. People also get discouraged when they have prayed for a sick loved one, or for some other purpose to be fulfilled in their lives, only to have the individual die, or the purpose not actualized. When this happens, the resulting frustration and discouragement are understandable, but don't stop praying. Look at the lack of fulfillment from a different point of view. Don't punish yourself because you think you may have done something wrong to deserve the bad situation, nor think God has failed you.

Most people want God to meet their needs and respond to their individual requests, but such requests, seen from a different perspective, may not be in the best interest of all who are affected by it. As an example, think about what the world would be like if all the dying people being prayed for survived? From another perspective, certain answers to prayer may not be possible, or even helpful, or in our best interest. How many times have you wished for something that you didn't get or didn't do, and later realized that you're glad that wish didn't come true?

Keep your heart and mind open to the faith that the universe is good, that you are in the right place at the right time, and that the goodness within you will unfold in perfect harmony with God's goodness. The most useful prayer in difficult situations is to pray for God's will to be done and then trust that whatever that might be is the best solution to the situation. By the way, who do we think we are to assume we know what is best? I believe that it is wiser to give that responsibility to God and to trust that the outcome will be good.

The universe is not arbitrary, it is good. Most people have a hard time understanding why bad things happen to good people. Some might think that a person deserves what he gets out of life. Good people live the good life and the bad are left behind. Some people actually think that they are not good enough to receive the abundance that is present in the world. I completely disagree. We all deserve the good that is in us and in our universe. We need to remember that all things are working toward our good, and we are working with them in the light of the wisdom and power of the universe.

Prayer is a type of energy. Some people think that prayer is energy, but there is no evidence that it is. Prayer does not follow the physical laws of energy as we understand them today. Energy weakens as it travels from its source. Prayer does not. There is no relationship to proximity of the prayed-for object or person and the praying person. Prayer has the same effect from two feet away as it does from the other side of the world.

Prayer doesn't follow the classic laws of physics. To understand how prayer does work, we need to expand our concepts of reality. Einstein, commenting on the clockwork type of physics that brought man to the moon, said, "The significant problems we face [today] cannot be solved by the same level of thinking that created them." Likewise, we need a new paradigm in physics to understand how prayer affects our lives.

Historian Arnold Toynbee put the same thought another way in his challenge-response formula, "When the response is equal to or surpasses the challenge . . . [we] call it success. As soon as the challenge changes, the old once-successful response is no longer successful. Thus nothing fails like success." In other words, our usual response of trying harder by increasing the frequency or intensity of what we have done in the past will not work when confronted with new challenges. (An interesting definition of insanity is someone who continues to respond in the same unsuccessful way to a stimulus or situation.) Are you ready to change the way you think and approach problems? Here are a few sentence stems to try.

When I am frustrated, I . . .

When I hear a new idea, I . . .

I try new ways to do . . .

During my pregnancy, I will . . .

There are many things in our lives that we accept on faith without a full understanding of how they work. Penicillin is a good example. When it was discovered, medical scientists knew it cured infections like pneumonia, but they did not know why. Nurse-midwives in Vienna in the late 1800s washed their hands between delivering their patients, and they had fewer maternal deaths. They did not understand the germ theory at the time, but eventually everyone started washing before delivering babies.

Even television is an interesting example. I suspect most of us don't fully understand how it works, but when we sit down to watch the evening news, we know that it will be there on our favorite channel. So, let's accept that prayer works, even though we cannot explain it. It may change the shape and rhythm of the neuropeptide receptors on the surfaces of our body's cells, which makes them more susceptible to the effects of our positive neuropeptides.

Your Mind Is Bigger Than You Think

I'll talk in depth about prayer in a few pages, but first I want you to ponder the possibility that your mind extends beyond your body. Traditionally in Western cultures, we envision our minds residing in our brains and affecting only our bodies. Not so.

I am sure you can you relate to some experiences that I've had. Pulling up to a stoplight in my car, having the feeling that someone was staring at me, and then turning my head to catch them in the act of looking right at me. How about a phone ringing and knowing instantly who is calling; or thinking about a person and having them arrive at the door; or sitting with someone and thinking about the same subject they ask about without any previous conversation on the topic? There is ample research that supports the concept that our minds extend beyond our bodies.

One study of college students showed that they could accurately indicate when another student was staring at their image on a TV monitor in a separate room. A similar study was done using a Galvanometer. A group of untrained college students affected the nervous tension, as measured by the Galvanometer, of another group of volunteers in a separate room, just by thinking about them being nervous, or imagining the needle of the Galvanometer moving in the direction indicating nervousness. I believe there is a suprahuman consciousness that we each can relate to, without the use of our five senses. This concept challenges traditional views and is not popular among my peers, but many cultures on Earth, other than those that developed in Europe, accept the concept that our bodies are mainly fields of energy, influenced by other energy forces, and that our minds extend well beyond our bodies. This is not foreign to the present-day thinking of physicists, who proved that atoms are mostly space filled with fields of energy.

We are much more than machines limited to the confines of our bodies. Humans in all cultures throughout history have intuitively felt connected to each other and to the universe. Do you feel this way? Think about it. It may help you to write endings to these sentence stems:

I believe that I am isolated and on my own because . . .

I feel connected to my loved ones when . . .

I think my mind extends beyond my body because . . .

I am loved by God because . . .

When I pray, my unborn child . . .

Discuss your sentence completions and thoughts with your infant's father, your life partner, and/or other loved ones. Ask them to do their own sentence stemming. Do their opinions surprise you? If you have major differences in your sentence endings, I strongly suggest you discuss them and come to a consensus, especially on this question about our relationship to all mankind and to the universe. What is their answer to Einstein's question about the universe being friendly to humans? Feeling safe will give you and your loved ones the confidence that you can handle this pregnancy, and you can work effectively as partners with health care providers to triumphantly conclude this pregnancy and birth a healthy and happy full-term infant.

The Experimental Evidence of Prayer Power

The excellent empirical scientific evidence that prayer is a powerfully effective force in our world was generated by multiple well-designed investigations using the most sophisticated scientific methods available. These studies clearly demonstrate that no particular religion or prayer technique produces results better than another, and that prayer is not just a matter of faith in God, but rather a power of love, empathy, and compassion.

Dr. Larry Dossey, an internist and respected medical researcher, describes the scientific evidence on prayer in his outstanding book *Healing Words: The Power of Prayer and the Practice of Medicine.*[2] The National Institutes of Health now has an Office of Alternative Medicine, which is conducting national research projects on this important subject.

The Objections to Prayer's Power

Some medical scientists think that the positive prayer studies are just due to a "file drawer" effect—if enough studies are done, then some positive results will occur solely by chance; and if all the negative studies were published, they would swamp the positive ones.

Dr. Robert Rosenthal of Harvard University is a scientist who has devoted most of his professional life to evaluating and studying controversial data of clinical research in such varied areas of study as parapsychology and psychology. He was commissioned by the National Research Council to evaluate the research on prayer. He gave prayer research high marks on quality and validity.[3]

In spite of this, the medical community still does not want to accept it. Most health care providers are leery of prayer. Their bias is that prayer is separate from science, and they have to think logically and analytically, which eliminates spirituality. They believe religion and medicine do not mix, therefore the results of these studies are not published in the prestigious, scientific medical journals. This disagreement between science and religion has been brewing for centuries, but the quality of recent scientific prayer research is helping us find a common ground of understanding.

Here are a few sentence stems:

I feel "heart connected" to my unborn child when . . .

I think prayer is . . .

My universe is . . .

God's plan for my pregnancy is . . .

World-class healers have known for years that the most important part of their healing process is to have empathy and compassion for their patients. Science is finally catching up.

Prayer works. Our minds go beyond our bodies. And God has the capacity to heal us. What is interesting is that spontaneous healings occur in people who are not trying to force God to heal them, but rather are passive and detached from their illness. They don't mind being healed, but they are not desperate. They believe that no matter what happens, they will be all right. The fate of their illness is up to a cosmic force—the universe or God—who is greater than themselves or the medical establishment. They don't aggressively go after positive visualization, nor take special vitamins, but rather they accept their illness and their possible pending death as a part of life.

Our marvelous bodies are designed to heal themselves. They are carefully engineered by evolutionary forces since the time living organisms appeared on earth to respond to threats in their environment. That is why we have such fantastic defense mechanisms to fight bacteria, viruses, and cancer. Defense cells in our body recognize when other cells are not well. These cells are then attacked and destroyed. This ability has been carefully selected through the ages by our genes and passed on to each new generation. The problem comes when our minds interfere with our inherited self-healing system. Please trust that God has a marvelous plan working in your body, and all is working for the health of you and your unborn infant.

This lesson is taught well in the biofeedback laboratory, where people are trying to learn to meditate. Using biofeedback equipment they quickly learn that they cannot force a meditative state to lower their blood pressure and heart rate, but it spontaneously appears when they let go and just let it happen. The same is true when we go to sleep each night. Have you every tried to force yourself to sleep? No, of course not, you just let it happen. I think maybe the Beatles were on to something with their song "Let It Be."

A series of spontaneous remissions of stomach cancer in a group of patients—usually a fatal disease—has been reported in Japan. The one common psychological attitude in all of these cancer patients was their harmony with the reality of their illness. They became spiritually introspective and contemplative. They did not battle the cancer, nor take an aggressive psychological stance toward it, but rather, gave thanks for the experience, then stepped aside, and trusted the wisdom in a higher power. They learned how to be with the illness and to let go of its outcome. They were living the statement, "Thy will be done." Their lives, and the outcome of their situations, were lifted up to the wisdom of God—an important lesson we all need to learn.[4]

Beliefs

Your critical beliefs are fundamental to the welfare of your pregnancy. What you believe you are is important. What you believe about the universe being a safe place for you is important. What you believe about the competency of yourself, your support group, and your medical team is important. If these beliefs cause fear and stress, they can increase your stress neuropeptides that may affect the developing fetal brain.

There are different types of prayer. The first and most common is intercessory prayer, which is a call for help for someone in need. Prayer experiments demonstrate that people don't have to believe in prayer to receive the benefit of someone else's prayers. However, the beliefs of the people praying is very important in affecting the prayed-for people or things.

There are two types of intercessory prayers—directed and nondirected. Of the two, nondirected prayers seem to have the greater effect in the laboratory; because the praying person, believing in the wisdom of God, calls for the best possible potential in the situation to be manifested. The work of the Spindrift Organization on prayer effects in lower organisms found that nondirected praying was two to four times more effective than directed praying.[5]

A directed prayer is for a specific request, like carrying the pregnancy to term, and delivering a healthy and happy baby. That is an acceptable prayer, and one I encourage, particularly, if you have a strong belief in the power of praying. While you are praying a directed prayer, you also know in your heart that you are in a safe place, and that no matter the outcome of the pregnancy, you will be able to handle the situation and ultimately be all right. The Japanese cancer patients did not just resign themselves to their cancer and give up. They had a belief that no matter what the outcome of their illness, they would be all right because their higher power is good. Their own preferences did not get in the way. This is a quite different attitude from one of not caring and giving up. It is similar to the spiritual optimism expressed by Frankl's group in the Nazi concentration camps.

Another type of prayer is petitionary prayer, or a request for yourself. This type of prayer is strongly linked to beliefs, and is close to the placebo effect. It is best to put these prayers in the present tense and to use first-person pronouns much like the positive affirmations used to conquer your internal chatterbox. (See chapter 10, "Growing Beyond Your Fears.")

For me, the most powerful prayer is the nondirected petitionary prayer. It builds self-confidence and brings peace of mind that is priceless.

Some other types of prayer are prayers of gratitude and centering prayers, which I'll discuss in the section on meditation in chapter 19.

Use your journal now to complete these sentence stems:

I believe . . .

When I try and fail . . .

I pray when . . .

To me, spiritual optimism means . . .

Unfortunately, a lot of patients don't pay enough attention to what their health care providers believe. In chapter 18, which deals with selecting a health care professional, you will read about the importance of matching your beliefs and values with those of your caregivers. Their beliefs have a tremendous affect on your well-being, but I am amazed—and dismayed—at most patients' lack of attention to this powerful force at work in medicine.

Some of my colleagues pride themselves on being scientists; they try to be dispassionate, cool, and unemotional. They feel that they have to be this way in order to present a realistic, scientific picture of their patients' conditions, plus they believe it is the best way to make good clinical decisions. On the contrary, even a health care professional with no feelings is going to affect you. You need to decide if an aloof, detached attitude and a disbelief in prayer are going to adversely affect your pregnancy, or interfere with your relationship with your medical provider.

The best way to evaluate the effects of belief systems in your relationship with your providers is to be aware of how you feel when you are around them, and when you leave their office. Do you feel better or worse after seeing them? It's important to feel connected to your health care providers, and to feel good and uplifted after seeing them. You want them to accept you as you are, and to support your personal choices.

Do you find yourself keeping back some information about yourself from your health care providers? This is not a good situation for you or your unborn child. Don't be ashamed that you may have different beliefs from medical professionals. It is in your best interests to select one with whom you are comfortable, even if you don't share the same beliefs. Just find someone who at least respects and is comfortable with your spirituality.

A Harvard study that shows that one third of the population uses some type of alternative medicine while receiving care from their physician, and most keep it from their doctor, because they don't want him or her to know, and are afraid of being scolded.[6] That is not a good situation. If this study describes your relationship with your health care provider, then you should either confess it, or move on.

See what your results are when completing these sentence stems:

A visit to my health care provider makes me feel . . .

My health care provider believes . . .

Putting Prayer to Work for You

It makes sense to put prayer to work along with modern medical technology. If you have a surgical condition, like the need for a C-section, then you need surgery, and all the drugs and technology that support that operation. But I contend that you will have a quicker recovery and better results if you and your loved ones pray during your operation and recovery.

Do you intellectually accept that it is a good idea to pray, but the act of praying seems foreign or uncomfortable? Don't get hung up on this point. If you need to pray, "just do it," as they say in the television commercials. If it helps you to put on tennis shoes, as that commercial proposes, that's okay. Trust your instincts; you will be doing it right. Prayer has been a natural act for men and women for a long time, and there is nothing fancy about it. I suggest you open each fetal love break with a nondirected petitionary prayer. I can feel such prayers change my neuropeptide mix. With practice and faith you will be sending fetal love messages of spiritual optimism and unconditional love to your unborn child—a wonderful gift to both you and your developing baby.

There is an interesting old Islamic tale related in Dr. Dossey's book. A poor old man lives very humbly with his son, and their prized possession, a horse, runs away. The men in the village come to visit and sympathetically say to the old man, "Too bad your horse ran away." The old man responds, "Perhaps." The next day the horse returns leading a beautiful black stallion, and the neighbors return to congratulate the old man on his wonderful fortune and he replies, "Perhaps." The next day the son, trying to train the majestic stallion, breaks his leg. The neighbors give sympathy and the old man gives his usual response, "Perhaps." The following week the army rides into their village looking for conscripts and they pass by his son with the broken leg.

The wonderful lesson of the story is not to place too much significance on the ups and downs of day-to-day life. It is wiser to take a long-term perspective, to say that no matter what happens today, you will be all right because your universe is safe. You will have ups and downs during your pregnancy. Some days you will have energy, others none. Some days you will feel happy, others not. Some visits to your care provider will be encouraging, others possibly distressing. When you are in these varying experiences, remember the old man's sentiment and response to his fellow villagers.

Most of us think we need to be assertive if we want to improve our situation. We tend to attack our problems. But prayer is more of a state of *being* than a skill of *doing*. How you pray is not as important as what you feel while you are praying. Just remember the importance of compassion, empathy, and love. Find your own way, be adventuresome, do what feels authentic. Admit your needs. This is not easy, but it is essential. The first step in prayer is developing a relationship with God. This means being candidly honest. It is easy to start prayers with an "I need" statement. It is far better to trust that the best outcome of the situation is unfolding, and like the old man in the Islamic story, our role is to keep tuned in, stay levelheaded, and just let it be.

Here are a few sentence stems:

When I pray, I . . .

What I need is . . .

Since pregnant, I am . . .

Love

Love is important to you, your partner, and to your unborn child, but what exactly is love? During the early 1940s a study was conducted in an orphanage where the children were divided into two groups. They both received the same nutritional and custodial care, but the group that had more human contact and received love and attention grew faster, had fewer infections, and one half the death rate of the children who were not nurtured. Without love infants die.

Prayer correlates with love, not religion. Even an agnostic who does not believe in God can produce a prayer effect, if he is capable of loving the prayer object. I believe that God is loving and is always ready to forgive me for all my mistakes. I did not earn this love—it is simply a blessing for me to receive. At times this seems too easy, because I think I don't deserve it; therefore I don't trust it. Everything else in my life I have earned or worked for, but God's love is just there for me to take!

Love is also important to your health, and the health of your fetus. Science shows that the richer our social relationships and the more empathetic we are, the lower the death rates due to illnesses, including heart disease. Research has demonstrated that men who were in loving relationships had a 50 percent lower incidence of angina. Prayer with love alters our minds and changes our bodies.

An interesting result of an experiment was reported in the journal *Science,* one of the world's most prestigious scientific journals. A group of rabbits were fed different diets to see what effect it would have on their cholesterol metabolism and the formation of arterial plaques, the main cause of cardiovascular disease. The scientists kept getting a response that was difficult to understand. The rabbits in the lower cages in the animal lab consistently developed fewer cholesterol plaques in their arteries regardless of the diet they received.

They finally realized that the laboratory technician—who was short—was taking the rabbits out of the lower cages to play with them during her hours off work. They redesigned the study to look at the effect of fondling on the plaque formation, and they discovered that the rabbits that received more loving attention had less disease. Before being published, this study was repeated three times with the same results—love heals!

Most people think of love as a feeling, but it is simply a choice. You can choose to love regardless of the conditions of what happens, or what people do to you. Remember Frankl's group of prisoners who choose spiritual optimism in the face of a Nazi concentration camp.

Popular songs and movies falsely present romance as love. Romance is certainly more exciting and interesting than love, but it is not nearly as important. Romance is a feeling produced by our body's neuroendocrine system when we become physically or psychologically attracted to someone. It is best described as enmeshment—a feeling of oneness with the other that gives each the sense of wholeness and unity. I prefer to think of this feeling as horniness—to have sex and procreate so the human species can survive—a feeling far different from love.

What is important for you and your partner to realize is that this feeling will not last forever, and soon after the urge to merge appears, the boundaries between your identities will snap back into place. The relationship may or may not survive the reestablishment of the identity boundaries, but this is when the work of love begins.

Love is different from enmeshment. It is the willingness to work on behalf of the other's interest. This does not mean to work for what you think is their best interest, but rather to work for what your love partner thinks is his or her best interest.

Being a member of a pregnant family is one of life's most loving situations. There is something magical about another life growing and developing in us that creates new awareness of our importance to each other and to our unborn child. The realization that the choices you make will affect your unborn infant is a powerful motivator to evaluate and change lifelong behaviors. Pregnancy opens our minds and hearts to new information and new ways of living and caring for each other.

Love gives us the power to change thoughts and behaviors that may adversely affect our lives and the pregnancy. Once the child is delivered, the power of love continues; and for many of us this is the first time we fully understand the difference between romance and love. The strong bond between parents and their newborn infant empowers parents to work and sacrifice for the welfare of their child.

And that is the true meaning of love.

Please finish up this chapter now by completing these sentence stems:

Now I believe . . .

Now I will pray . . .

My universe is . . .

For me love is . . .

After finishing the last set of sentence stems, review the ones earlier in the chapter and compare the insights that developed while doing these exercises. You may want to discuss these last two chapters with family members whose faith you trust and respect or with a religious counselor.

$\mathcal{G}$rowing Beyond Your Fears

There is no fear in love; but perfect love casts out fear.
—*1 John 4:18*

Love is what we were born with. Fear is what we learned here.
—*Marianne Williamson*

How many times has fear stopped you from doing something you wanted or needed to do? Fear can literally stop us in our tracks, impede our growth, and block accomplishments. If we succumb to its power, we will never grow materially, psychologically, or spiritually. We all have fears; some instinctual ones like acrophobia (the fear of being in high places) we're born with. They are important to our safety, health, and happiness. Others, like fear of snakes, are learned. They are inappropriate and inhibit our lives.

Learned fears keep us from fully participating in life and achieving our goals. They keep us in a comfort zone where we achieve little because we risk nothing. We are far more comfortable in our daily routines with the same behaviors, going to the same jobs, and not thinking about new, better, more rewarding ways to live.

How different would your life be without your fears? Write down the things you would do differently if you lived without fear. Would you be in your same job? Would you still live in the same location? Would you have accomplished more in your life?

Write the endings to the following sentence stems in your journal.

If I had only one month to live, I would . . .

If I inherited all the money I could possibly need, I would . . .

If I knew that I would not fail, I would . . .

Most of us would do things differently if we knew that we didn't have to worry about the future, finances, or failures. Unfortunately, many of us bring the fears we learned from the past and project them into our future, which keeps us in our limiting comfort zone where we think there is less risk. Psychologists claim that all the goals you listed in the above sentence stems are possible if you control your fears. In fact, you are likely to be successful in precisely the areas you listed above because they reflect your innate talents, which can bring you happiness and rewards.

Feel the Fear and Just Do It

Fear is certainly part of being pregnant. We all have concerns about the health of the developing fetus and our family's future. Let's look at some of the problems that can develop in pregnancy that you and/or your life partner can learn to control.

Knowledge is power, and empowerment increases your ability to control risks and improve the outcome of your pregnancy. If we felt confident that we could handle anything that comes our way, we would have no fears. The simple truth is that all you have to do to reduce your fears is to increase your confidence that you can handle whatever comes your way, such as delivering a baby, raising a family, and being a parent.

Psychologist Susan Jeffers, Ph.D., describes five truths about fear in her book *Feel the Fear and Do It Anyway.* Here are some of the points she makes.[1]

- Fear will always be a part of your life as long as you continue to grow and stretch your capabilities to accomplish new goals, to actualize your dreams. For you, this may currently be birthing a healthy baby and creating a loving family.

- The only way to get rid of the fear of doing something and feeling better about yourself is to go out and do it while squarely facing the fear. Fear of a particular situation usually dissipates when it is confronted. You will have more confidence in facing your fears of pregnancy as you experience the actual events, with the added bonus of increased self-confidence.

- You are not the only one who feels fear when doing something new. All of the people who look and act so confident when taking on new challenges are really frightened. The secret is to move through the event while feeling the fear, then the fact that you are afraid becomes irrelevant.

- Pushing through the fear while you experience it is less frightening than living with the underlying fear of not doing it and feeling helpless. The more helpless you feel, the more frightened you become. If you become obsessed with the dreadful "what if" catastrophes of life, you will take fewer and fewer risks until you become paralyzed with fear.

"What if" are the two most loaded words in the English language. They can create disaster out of any situation because they force us to think of negative rather than positive outcomes. If you are troubled by "what if" scenarios, write them down and actively think about the positive "what if" outcomes. This will at least balance your thinking.

Take a moment now to write down your "what if"s. Start by writing one of your fears at the top of each page and on the next line write "What if." Then list all the bad possibilities associated with each fear. Think deeply to be sure you get all your fears down on paper. You will learn that once the fears are on paper they don't seem as formidable, and are worth the risk to pursue your dreams. Think about which fears are stopping you from achieving your dream. Is it really stopping you from doing it or is there another fear?

Now, turn the page and write your hopes and dreams on the top of the next few pages and repeat the process. During this exercise the "what if"s will be more positive and should elicit excitement. These are your dreams, and you can make them come true. Be sure to share these exercises with your life partner. He can be a great resource for encouragement, particularly if he knows your dreams and what is keeping you from achieving them.

The Origins of Our Fears

Where do our fears come from? Psychologists tell us that they are communicated to us from our parents and other influential people during early childhood. They are based on these childhood stories, which we play over and over in our minds until we become conditioned to respond with fear whenever that memory or similar situation appears in our minds or in real life.

Can you remember times when your parents told you to be careful as you left the house? I was well into my forties when my dad was still telling me to be careful, and to watch out for whatever worried him at the time. Can you remember your parents ever telling you to "take some risks today" as you went out to play? Of course not. They were probably constantly telling you to "be careful," which carries the double message—not only is the world dangerous but, more important from the psychological viewpoint, you are unable to handle it.

This powerful message instilled in your developing psyche the fear that you cannot handle life's events. These messages are like software that drives our decisions and emotions well into our senior years. How much better if we made life decisions based on love, our hopes and dreams, and a feeling of being connected to God, rather than on fear and isolation. Psychology has proved that we make better decisions when they are based on positive goals and we feel safe.

Many of our fears are based on a belief system we are so enmeshed in that we don't even perceive it. It's like fish asking each other, "What is this water that everyone is talking about?" They are immersed in the sea and have never experienced anything else but water. They don't even know it exists—and so it is with many of our fears. The best way to correct this is to get them on paper using the above exercises and discuss the results with your life partner. Think of the worst possible outcome of the action you fear, and then decide if it is worth the risk. When I do this, I realize that many of my fears are unrealistic and the worst possible outcome doesn't justify the worry. Try it and see if this is also true for you.

Here are a few sentence stems.

If I believed that God was good . . .

If I believed I was good enough, I . . .

Discovering Your Beliefs Behind Fear

Sometimes it is difficult to discover our beliefs until we are confronted by new information or a new situation. Most of us are afraid of heights, but we didn't know it until we were put in a situation that provoked the fear. Some people are able to overcome their fears to enjoy life more; many technical rock climbers tell about their fear of heights before they got involved in the sport. My own son enjoyed the excitement of facing his fears. Some people get so high on facing fear that they participate in "extreme sports." I'm not suggesting that we all become extreme skiers, technical rock climbers, or free-fall parachuters. What I am suggesting is that it is very rewarding to overcome fear. It's a builder of self-confidence.

The fear of physical dangers like heights and snakes is a type of fear that I think is easier to manage than the psychological fears that can be more damaging to our future. A common psychological fear is the fear of intimacy. Are you willing to share all your thoughts with your life partner? Sometimes the more important the person is to our happiness, the more difficult it is to tell the truth. We think that by not being completely frank about our thoughts and feelings we are helping the relationship. This is not true, and overcoming the fear of truth telling is important to your relationship not only with your life partner, but also with your children. Please do now the "what if" exercise on your fear of truth telling with your life partner. I discuss how to work on this in part 3.

We commonly call new situations or new information a "crisis." The Chinese word for crisis is made of two syllables. One means danger, and the other opportunity. How do you respond to the crises in your life? Do you see them as opportunities, or filled only with danger? Can you honestly answer Einstein's question, "Is the universe a safe place"? The mental messages you send yourself during crises or times of stress are vital to your health and the health of your fetus.

Please complete the following sentence stems.

When I was a child, I was afraid of . . .

When I suspect there is danger, I . . .

I like myself least when . . .

Looking back over my life I can hardly believe that at one time I . . .

It is not easy for me to admit . . .

The activities in my life that have meaning are . . .

I like myself the most when . . .

When I am in a new situation or place, I . . .

I believe the universe is safe, so when I . . .

Stress-Hardy People

An excellent psychological study about stress-hardy businesspeople whose jobs were threatened by the divestiture of their corporation found that some businesspeople become frightened and fold, while others seem to thrive on the stress of the situation. People who thrive have three basic qualities. They possess a strong commitment to the corporation and appreciate the value their jobs brought to it. They view their work as having meaning and purpose, and they usually express love for their work and want to continue to work in spite of the stress. They are able to do this because they see the change as a challenge or opportunity, rather than one of danger and despair.

These stress-hardy individuals also have a sense of control. They know that they cannot always control the life events around them, but they are confident that they can control their attitude and response to these events. They know what they can and cannot do about the situation. They know when to hold on, and when to let go. The quality of being stress-hardy is nicely summed up in the serenity prayer of Alcoholic Anonymous, which says, "God, give me the serenity to accept the things I cannot change, the courage to change the things I can, and the wisdom to know the difference."

To become a stress-hardy person, you must have a strong belief system that assures you that you can handle the situation. This requires faith based on a strong foundation, which allows us to remain flexible and open to new experiences and possibilities. In order to do this, you must feel safe and have the ability to confidently and enthusiastically say "yes" to your universe. This is one reason why spirituality and/or religion is so important to the quality of life. You cannot feel safe without it. To feel safe you must believe in a power greater than yourself, a power that is loving and forgiving.

Review the last two sentence stems in the above exercise to evaluate your degree of stress hardiness. If you need improvement in this area, then please begin working on your spirituality by talking with a friend you feel is well developed spiritually or with a spiritual counselor. This is important fetal love work for both you and your unborn child.

Managing Fear

How many times have you feared doing something only to find that the experience was not so frightening when it was over? Most of us have lived for so long with our fears, that we have problems giving them up. We are certain that most of them are caused by the people and dangers around us. We think that if conditions would just change, our fears would disappear. But our fears are based on how we choose to interpret both the past and present events of our daily lives, and not on what we actually experience. We have the misconception that our fears protect us. Does the fear of heights protect the technical mountain climber? No! What protects rock climbers is respect for the safety aspects of their sport and a sound understanding of their skill level. Their fear only prevented them from enjoying their sport until they climbed while facing it.

These acquired fears, such as fear of snakes, can be effectively treated by systematically desensitizing the individual. This is done by relaxing the patient, while gradually increasing the more frightening aspects of the fear. For example, a person frightened by snakes will first imagine being near a snake, seeing it, handling it, then look at pictures of the same sequence, and then physically experience the sequence, which ends with handling a live snake. This desensitization therapy is quite successful and is commonly done by behavior modification therapists.

We are afraid because we have been conditioned to live fearfully. The same event, such as a summer thunderstorm, will frighten one person, and offer a glorious display of nature's power to another who has not had the same conditioning. These two individuals have both experienced the same storm, but have completely different reactions to it.

Conditioning tends to run in families. A fearful person will always find something to fear, because he has been carefully taught to be afraid. Remember that you share your emotions with your unborn child via the neuroendocrine system. Your chronic fears and anxieties, if not recognized and properly managed, set the emotional tone of your unborn child, which can last a lifetime. It is far easier to prevent this from happening prenatally than it is to correct at school age.

Growing Beyond Fear

Some of the fears that we had as children are actually life-threatening, but as we grow older and became more self-sufficient, the reality of the fears diminish. For example, for an infant, the loss of love is a life-or-death situation, but for adults it is not as detrimental.

The studies done in the 1940s on infants in foundling homes demonstrated how important human contact was for the infants' survival. One group of infants received food, body care, and frequent loving contact with the caretakers. Another group of similar infants received the same diet and body care without the human contact. They did not receive the nurturing love. There was no one for them to bond to, to relate to, or to mirror their existence. Because of this experience, their pituitary glands, located at the base of the brain, did not produce growth hormones, and these infants withered away, in spite of adequate nutrition. Most of them died before they reached toddler age. Those who survived were emotionally damaged. They could not bond with other people and usually developed into sociopathic adults capable of stealing, maiming, and killing without guilt.

The same emotional isolation experienced by an adult will not present the same detrimental effects to his life and welfare, because the adult is more capable of handling the seclusion. He has a wider perspective of his experiences that helps him evaluate his fear reaction. His brain is less plastic, so its architecture is less likely to be changed by these negative experiences.

What about the common experience of a child who fears monsters in the closet or under the bed at night, which she perceives as threats to her safety? Pediatricians now recommend that families take their frightened child on a tour of her room and closets so she can face her imagined monsters. Once experienced, the child learns that she can handle the situation. She experienced the fear, went on the tour to face it, and learned that pushing through fear is less frightening than living with it. Most children will then happily and confidently fall asleep.

When we face physical danger, fear is not bad. It gives us energy and courage to fight for survival. Our hearts race, our breath quickens, and we develop superhuman strength, as neuropeptides like noradrenaline rush into our bloodstream to shift our metabolism into the work mode by pumping sugar and oxygen into our muscle cells. If we exert energy and consume the oxygen and sugar, and degrade the released hormones, there is no harm to our bodies; but, if we live in a chronic fear state, the neuropeptide surge and work-mode metabolism remain static, and damage our health and that of the unborn child.

We would never leave our cars on high idle with the parking brake on. It would cause undue wear and tear on the engine and other parts of the car. Instead, we turn the ignition off and rest the motor, allowing the engine to cool down. Like the automobile, our bodies in constant work mode with no physical activity will be adversely affected. We need to learn how to psychologically manage our fears, to turn off the metabolic response to them, and let our bodies recover, to lower the set points of our feedback loops for stress neuropeptides.

It's natural to have fears about the outcome of your pregnancy, or about the pain of labor and birthing. The key to breaking the habit of living fearfully is to become aware of your fears, and then make choices to change your thinking about them. I am here to help as your trailblazer, but the commitment and follow-through are your responsibility. Do you want to continue making decisions based on fears, to continue life as a fear victim, or do you want to change your thinking, and learn some new habits? The choice is yours.

The First Step: Take Charge of Your Chatterbox!

Taking responsibility for correcting your fears means controlling your biggest enemy—your chatterbox, the little voice in our mind that drives us all crazy, heralding gloom and doom. You may be so used to that voice that you aren't even aware of its presence, but we are all victims of it. Fortunately, there are effective ways of changing your chatterbox into a nurturing, loving voice. People don't like hanging out with enemies; so make your chatterbox a friend. It will change your life. You will begin enjoying being alone more. You will become happier and healthier, and your unborn child will benefit from the flow of positive neurotransmitters across the placenta.

To move from the pain of fear to a position of power over fear, you need to get in touch with your inner wisdom, which is powerful and loving, unlike your chatterbox. Do you see yourself as a victim, or are you taking responsibility for what happens in your life? Write your answer to this question now before going on with the rest of this chapter. Try these sentence stems:

I feel fear when . . .

I am a victim of . . .

I feel inadequate when . . .

How could God love me when I . . .

Taking responsibility for your life requires choosing your thought patterns. This may sound easy, but it is not. It takes work, consistent practice, and patience. It's a skill that can be learned, and is one of the most powerful gifts you can give yourself and your unborn child.

So many people think that circumstances or other people cause their fears and explain why they are in the present situation. If we see ourself as a victim, we move from a position of power into pain and paralysis. Being a victim means giving away your power. No one can control the events around their lives, but each of us controls our reaction to the circumstances around us. No one can take away our feelings, the meaning of our lives, the attitude we choose to take into each situation. Remember the spiritual optimism of Dr. Frankl's group in the Nazi prison camps.

You can live more powerfully by taking responsibility for your life. Never blame someone else for what you are feeling, doing, or experiencing. You are solely responsible for what is going on in your head. If something is not working right in your life, then ask yourself, How can I change it? Try an experiment of going one week without complaining about circumstances or criticizing anyone.

Taking responsibility for your life doesn't mean blaming yourself. Don't make yourself a victim of your circumstances. This may sound contradictory, but it's not. Understand that you may have fears based on past experiences, but while you were learning to fear, you were doing the best you could in those circumstances. You may have had painful experiences in a medical office, or in a hospital, and these memories of pain and discomfort bring back your fear response.

Now things are different. You are learning new ways to think, and your past experiences can be put into a new perspective. You are not the same person you were years ago. You are not even the same as you were moments ago. Your life is like the river that passes by the shore—there is a continuous flow of new and different water, just as there is a continuous flow of experience in your life constantly presenting new opportunities. Learning new ways to think and react to life will take time. Be patient and know you can do it.

The first step is to learn when and where you are presently not taking responsibility in your life, so you can change. Find the places in your life where you are taking the role of the victim. Pay attention to what you complain about. When do you feel fear, anger, pain, self-pity, envy, impatience, or helplessness? Take note of when these emotions arise, and try to find the reasons for them. Pay attention to your feelings, and ask, Why am I feeling this way? Review the previous sentence stems you completed and then try these new ones using the above negative emotions in the blank space: I feel . . . when . . . This is a great way to explore what effect blame is having in your life. I highly recommend it. This is a difficult exercise, but well worth the effort. Think of it as fetal love work for your unborn child.

When you complain, you are not taking responsibility for your happiness, but rather blaming someone or something else for it, and this gives away your choice to be happy. There is only one person in the world who can make you happy or unhappy, and that is you. With this realization, you can start taking better care of yourself and become more self-nurturing.

Positive Thinking Is Realistic

Positive thinking is a buzzword from pop psychology. My dad tried to get me to think positively about homework when I was in grade school. I thought it was the most ridiculous concept on the face of the earth. How could I pass a test on material I did not understand just by saying, "I am a smart student"? The reality was that I had to study and understand the material in order to make a good grade.

What I didn't know how to do then but now practice on a daily basis is to adjust my thinking to help me understand and remember new material. Before studying something new, I spend a few minutes relaxing and getting my mind focused on the task. I visualize myself using the new information in ways that benefit me and/or my patients. I give myself a mental reward before starting the difficult task.

Next, I write what I already know about the subject before reading new information. This helps me relate the new material to what I already know and I can retain it better.

Preparing to study with a positive affirmation is an excellent learning skill. If I had done that in grade school, I would have been a better student. On the other hand, if I knew the material well, and then told myself that I was not going to get a good grade because I was stupid and did not test well, I would fail the test no matter how well I knew the material. See the difference? It is subtle but important.

Today, an expanding branch of modern psychology called neurolinguistics verifies the importance of the internal chatterbox in our lives. So, my dad was right after all.

But one caution about positive thinking. Don't use it as an excuse to avoid reality. No one is immune to pain, and positive thinking should not be used to deny it. Life is painful, yet most of us spend enormous amounts time and energy trying to avoid pain. This is futile. There is no way to avoid it. It is much wiser to accept pain as part of life and realize it often leads to spiritual and psychological growth. Our task is to find the positive meaning in trying life situations.

Positive thinking is a difficult concept. Most people think it is unrealistic, but why do we assume that negative thinking is more realistic than positive thinking? We automatically assume that our negative suppositions are realistic, while the positive ones are not. We expect bad outcomes to occur and constantly worry about them. Research has shown that over 90 percent of what we worry about never occurs. Worrying is just so much wasted energy.

So, make the commitment to work on your chatterbox. The work will improve the outcome of your pregnancy—in fact, it is likely to be more important than the prenatal vitamins you are taking. Positive thinking also increases the comfort and welfare of your developing fetus by washing it with positive neurotransmitters (see part 1).

Here's an experiment in positive thinking you can try. Ask your life partner to extend his right arm in front of him and make a fist. Ask him to resist your attempts to push it down. Usually you cannot budge the arm down. Now ask him to close his eyes and repeat the words, "I am weak and an unworthy person" ten times aloud with conviction. Have him open his eyes, extend his fist in front of him, and you try again to push it down. Most of the time he will not be able to resist your pushing to the same extent as the first time. Now ask him to close his eyes again and repeat ten times, "I am strong and a worthy person." Repeat the arm pushing, and you will see that his strength comes back just by changing the content of the words he used.

This amazing demonstration shows that words are powerful in affecting our unconscious minds. It doesn't matter if we believe the words or not, because our unconscious minds don't judge them for accuracy yet they still affect our bodies. Our minds just receive the message, and the arm becomes weaker or stronger. Our minds do control our bodies, so you can see how important it is for us to feed our minds the right words. When you do, you will act differently and, in turn, the world will perceive you differently and treat you differently.

To turn negative thoughts that steal your power into positive, empowering ones, do the same things you would if you were starting an exercise program to get into shape. Instead of strengthening your muscles, you will be strengthening your mind through discipline, commitment, and practice—the ingredients for all human progress (see part 3).

After the training, you will need to continue a maintenance program, which will be easier because of the positive feedback you'll receive. The hard part of any new behavior is getting started and sticking with the routine long enough for it to become a habit. Most new habits can be developed after twenty days of practice. That's not long, so make the commitment now to go for it!

Developing a Mental Training Program

First, get a small cassette tape player and pick up some inspirational and motivational musical tapes. The science of music therapy is just emerging in this country, but it has long been used in Europe and particularly in the former Soviet bloc. Different types of music have different effects on brain metabolism and you want to look for music that helps relaxation and concentration.

In their book *Superlearning 2000,* Sheila Ostrander and Lynn Schroeder suggest the use of slow Baroque music played primarily with low-frequency instruments like the cello, violin, or guitar for alert relaxation. Their book is filled with scientific studies on the biological effect music has on the mind and how it enhances learning and concentration.[2]

For example, slow Baroque music played at 60 to 64 beats per minute in 4/4 time is the most effective for learning. They suggest the "Winter" movement from Vivaldi's *The Four Seasons,* and the Largo from his Concerto in D Major for guitar and strings. They found that acid rock and rap music drains the body of energy and suggest that one stay away from it. Even plants were adversely affected by it.

Next, start using affirmations. Write some positive quotes and affirmations on cards and put them where you can frequently see them. When you come across one of your cards, relax, and repeat it ten times aloud to yourself.

Writing an affirmation that will program your subconscious takes some special thought. Always make such statements positively, and put them in the present tense. As an example, the affirmation "I am powerful and loving" is much more effective than "I am no longer weak and afraid." A good place to find many wonderful affirmations is in Proverbs and the Song of Solomon in the Bible.

Earlier, I discussed the two most loaded words in the English language: "What if." I asked you to write down all of your "what if" scenarios in your journal, and then to think about some positive "what if" outcomes. Refer back to them now and let's see how to turn the negative ones around.

Remember, you are trying to change your flow of thoughts. Most "what if" scenarios are negative. I'd like you to stop feeling separate or alone, and come into a new reality of feeling safe with the oneness of the universe. Look for the good in people and situations. Think of yourself as being in the correct place for this time in your life, and remember that it was a long sequence of choices you made that has brought you here. By changing the choices from now on, you can bring yourself to a better place in your life.

What if you are not alone, but are really a small but significant part of a large supraconsciousness that is loving and supportive? Like the waves of the ocean, you are unique but part of the whole, which is good and nurturing. What if you are not expendable, but are precious, with unique talents meant for the grand development of the universe?

Your role as a child of the universe is just as important and precious as any other in the grand scheme of the evolving cosmic plan. From one perspective, some members of society appear to be more important than others, but from a different viewpoint this may not be true—in fact, it probably is not. Who would have thought that a simple O ring, a common washer that we all know and use on a daily basis, could have caused the space shuttle *Challenger* disaster? Yet it did.

Never underestimate your importance. No one else knows how important you are and what potential you possess. Like the pebble dropped in the quiet pool of water, our simple everyday thoughts and actions have ripple effects that are magnified as they expand ever outward. What if you did not have to search for meaning in your life? What if you knew with every fiber of your being that the purpose of your life is to love, and in return you are loved, and through this love you will find peace, and through peace you will understand God as seen in others and yourself?

What if this realization of finding love were as simple as not judging yourself, others, and situations? What if you are worthy for just being you and not for what you are doing or have done in the past? What if the act of forgiveness would free you to listen to the affirmations you have written so they will take hold of your soul and live in your heart forever?

Judgments are based on fear. Love is letting go of fear. By understanding fear we can let go of judgments and through forgiveness find peace and joy. What if the situations in your life that cause the most frustration and grief are presented to you as opportunities to learn about fear, forgiveness, and love? What if Joseph Campbell's conclusion is right, that myths teach us that in the darkest moments of our lives we are most likely to learn our most important lessons? What if the things that seem so unfair in our lives turn out to make sense many years later, when we are able to see them from a different perspective? What if all the help you need to change your life is available to you now and all you have to do is ask and it will be given to you?

All of these seemingly impossible beliefs are fervently embraced by millions of people. The reasons for their popularity is that they are true, and they work to improve the believers' lives. A study of the world's religions, which have remained with us for centuries, all support the above "what if" questions. What a great list of affirmations for you to use to change your life, as have million of others.

Once you have selected your affirmations and have written them down as described on cards, gather them together and record them in your own voice with the selected music in the background. Adjust the volume on the background music so your recording is mainly music and you have to pay close attention to hear your own voice recite the affirmations. This tape will become an excellent source of strength for you and your baby during your pregnancy.

In review, the goal is to out talk your negative chatterbox. This doesn't take extra time from your busy schedule. It just takes your becoming aware of the negative chatter, and replacing it with affirmations. Wake up in the morning and turn on the tape machine and listen to one side of the inspirational tape. When you first see yourself in the mirror, smile, and look behind your eyes into the soul of your mind. Don't be critical of what you see, just look with deep respect at the goodness within you. Say to yourself, "I am creating a beautiful day today." Watch carefully as you see your eyes change into a subtle smile. Feel the goodness within you, and let your light of virtue shine forth.

As you move through your morning routine, pay attention to the positive quotes you have placed in the places most likely to catch your eye—the bathroom mirror, the refrigerator door, your dresser, or the kitchen counter. As you dress, repeat your affirmations for at least ten minutes, always out talking your chatterbox. If you have an exercise routine, pump in some positive affirmations while you pump up your heart rate and respiration.

Make your car your temple of learning. Instead of listening to radio stations that produce popular music—I call it chewing gum for the brain—play music that lifts you up, or listen to an inspirational tape you have made. In your office, pay attention to the positive affirmations you have placed there. As pressures mount during the day, use your break times to give your brain positive energy by taking some deep cleansing breaths, using diaphragmatic breathing (see part 3 for more on this technique), while repeating your affirmations over and over, until the strength of your optimism comes back. Just remember to out talk your chatterbox. The positive messages you are sending your subconscious brain are new and it takes time to break old habits. When you come home, review your affirmation cards, and try to play some inspirational music just before going to sleep. Sleep reduces the conscious filters that block the flow of new information to the subconscious, so it is a great time to rescript the old tapes of negative thinking.

Committing to such a program will turn your world around. You'll start feeling better fairly soon, but that is not the time to stop doing it. This is a common mistake that people make when learning neurolinguistic techniques. Don't make the same one. Continue on, and you will have more energy, and be able to accomplish more than you imagined possible. You will laugh more, and attract positive people into your life, who will help reinforce your new behavior.

It's a good idea to tell everyone about the negative behaviors you are trying to stop so they can remind you if you fail to follow through. It is also a good idea to reveal your commitment to develop this new thought process only to the people who truly support your growth, because many friends who are not committed to your growth will use the information against your goal. They may not like the changes in you. They want you in their comfort zone. They don't have the courage, commitment, and energy that you have to break out of your comfort zone and into a new, better way of thinking, of gestating, and of birthing a healthy and happy baby.

Part III

*T*he Inner Journey to Parenting Your Unborn Child

11

Self-esteem: The Key to a Successful Pregnancy

Self-esteem isn't everything, it's just that there's nothing without it.
—Gloria Steinem

Life is filled with changes. Pregnancy is no exception. It changes your daily routines and places new demands on you like financial planning, buying new furniture and clothes, learning the demands of fetal brain development, and preparing for childbirth. These changes are only a few that we all face during our lifetimes. Although the changes you make are quite diverse, the process for creating them is the same. With adequate self-confidence, an attitude of being capable of doing things successfully, the prospect of making significant positive changes in your life improves. Self-confidence is only one part of self-esteem. So, let's get to work on building your self-esteem, which is so important to all aspects of life. It does not matter what level your self-esteem is, it can always be enhanced.

The primary reason for writing this book and spending so much time on the psychospiritual aspects of pregnancy is my firm conviction that you, and how well you manage the challenges of your pregnancy, are important to its outcome. With the help of your loved ones, you can manage the risks that determine the quality of your pregnancy better than we physicians can. How you think and what you believe about your abilities to do this greatly determine the success of your pregnancy. With faith and an understanding of the psychology of change, you will have the tools to accomplish the task of loving your unborn child to health and happiness.

The information in this book requires you to change some aspects of your thinking and/or behavior. Even if this pregnancy is risk free, and you are doing everything correct for your baby's welfare, you will face changes. Some pregnant couples don't understand the degree of change this milestone brings, until they take their baby home. They don't realize the demands of parenthood, and how it permeates every aspect of their lives, including their leisure time, their work, their finances, and their social activities. Next to the death of a spouse, pregnancy is the biggest life adjustment you will face.

The Importance of Self-esteem

What you think of yourself is the single most important judgment you make. It affects every aspect of your life: how high you will be promoted on the job, how well your marriage and other important relationships will develop, and how adeptly you will parent your child.

A low self-esteem is a self-fulfilling prophecy. If you don't feel that you are capable of handling the challenges of childbirth and childrearing, then you will most likely fail at meeting this important responsibility.

The income level of salespeople is a good example of the power of self-esteem. The salespeople who firmly believe that they are the best will have the higher incomes. The others will rise just to the level of their own estimates of self-worth. If for some reason a salesperson gets a higher than anticipated commission, he or she becomes disoriented and anxious and will subconsciously revert to his/her comfort zone of performance. This phenomenon is well studied and has been documented in the psychological literature.

Likewise, in business, many persons are promoted to the level of their incompetence. Most business managers think their subordinates' incompetence can be fixed with more training to develop job skills, but the root of the problem may not lie in the lack of job skills or intelligence, but rather in the employees' estimate of their capabilities, and whether they believe they deserve the promotion. If the employee does not think she is worthy of the promotion, she feels like an imposter when promoted.

The problem of poor self-esteem may seem like a terrible one with no solution, but I have shared with you Dr. Nathaniel Branden's technique of sentence stemming to help you achieve your goals. He has had years of experience in his private practice using this technique to raise people's self-esteem. This does not mean that it will be easy work. On the contrary, the work requires courage, dedication, and time. Pregnancy is a good opportunity to work on such major areas of self-help, and most pregnant families have the stamina to make large leaps in their spiritual and psychological growth as they prepare for parenting.

What is exciting about this fetal love work is that your self-esteem starts improving when you take that first step to change behaviors. Each step successfully completed builds a higher level of self-esteem, which helps your commitment to take the next step toward your goal. The way to make changes in your life is to change your thinking in small ways, which then changes your behavior.

Basic Concepts

There are some confusing misconceptions about self-esteem that need clarification. One is the idea that it is not good to have high self-esteem. Some think it is far better to be humble, because one is more likely to be successful. Actually, the reverse is true. The healthier your self-esteem, the more likely your success. The important distinction is that one can have a high self-esteem and still be modest. In fact, many arrogant personalities are a cover for a person's low self-esteem.

When I was young, I had this misconception about self-esteem. I don't know when it first started, but I do remember feeling uncomfortable when people gave me compliments. I felt like a fraud, because I thought I did not deserve them.

I also had the second and related burden of performing to meet people's expectations, because I thought that was the way to receive recognition and love. I had no sense of worth of my God-given endowments and could not recognize my talents, personality, intelligence, capacity to love, and integrity. I did not feel worthy of attention, affection, and love without achieving accomplishments others found laudable. If I failed to perform to the level of my or my loved ones' expectations, I feared I would lose their favor or love, a horrific predicament for a young man's developing psyche. This outwardly oriented concept of self-esteem was a heavy psychological burden that I carried all through my youth and early adulthood, well into my training as a physician. My self-esteem was performance based.

Most people like to receive compliments and gain notoriety, but that is not the basis of self-esteem. True self-esteem is based on how you think and feel about yourself. It is not based on how others think of you or on how well you perform on the job, in your relationships, or how popular you are with your friends. You may feel good when someone gives you a compliment, or you may feel guilty about accolades as I did while growing up, but self-esteem is not compliment based. The standards you set for this judgment need to be based on personal assessments of your past performance. This is different from accepting the standard of someone else's expectations.

That is why it is so important to have a faith system that verifies your value to yourself, regardless of your position in society, or how well you perform in any facet of your life. You need the confident belief that you are important to your developing baby, your life partner, your family and friends, and finally to the universe and God. What you are is more important than what you do, how you look, or who you are.

Dr. Robert Schuller, the pastor of the Crystal Cathedral, has spent his successful career preaching on biblical affirmations for our self-esteem. He uses the Bible as the basis for his teachings that God loves us, and we can change our lives by trusting in God's love and having the proper attitudes. Some people misinterpret the Bible as being punishing and filled with stories about God's revenge, when in reality the Bible affirms us as children of God, who loves us and accepts us for what we are.[1]

What You Are Is More Important Than Who You Are

Have you ever wondered why so many show business stars are so miserable when it appears that they have all that is needed to be happy? Why do they get into trouble with drugs and multiple broken relationships? Dr. Branden states that the reason for many superstars' failures is their lack of feeling genuine. They don't feel deserving of the adulation of their millions of fans. They feel phony and are afraid that if their true personalities were known, no one would like or admire them. They are living a fraudulent life, because they don't value themselves but rather a professional persona that is ephemeral. They may be popular and on top of the charts one week, but in the upcoming popularity poll they may falter, and if that should happen then their entire self-concept falls with their popularity rating.[2]

Genuine self-esteem is your estimate of your worth as a loving person who deserves happiness and your opinion about how capable you are of handling life's situations. Good self-esteem demands congruence between our thoughts and behaviors—we must openly express the self within. In this we can avoid living the life of an imposter with the constant fear of our true selves being revealed. Authentic living requires us to accept ourselves and to stop seeking to add value to our lives by faking the reality of what we are. This is not an easy task, and I will give you some action steps on how to do this in the section on living authentically.

We develop self-esteem by doing the required work to win the real battles in life. It takes courage and honesty to confront real life issues—like integrity. There is no quick fix, and it is not easy. There are no simple slogans that raise your self-esteem. There are many psychological programs on the market that claim to do so; but after reviewing the literature on this subject, I have come to the conclusion that sentence stemming is the best technique to use.

Like our hero on a quest, all growth requires leaving something behind and forging ahead into unknown territory that may be disorientating and uncomfortable. As you develop your self-esteem, you will leave your old comfortable way of thinking about yourself. This may cause some dramatic changes in your life, and in your relationship with your life partner and relatives. This quest, which takes stamina and courage, is similar to the quest facing your developing baby. Like you, she will birth into a new and unfamiliar environment. She will be separated from her supply of life sustenance and thrust into the unknown with the quick clip of your birth attendant's scissors cutting her umbilical cord. She will be forced to rely on new, untested capacities to sustain life and to continue her growth and development. As a neonatologist, I watch with amazement the deft adaptations babies make to life after birth. What your baby will face takes courage, stamina, and trust, an excellent example from which we can all learn.

You have already made major changes in your life. You have left your primary family, your school, and many of your school friends as you have grown and developed into an adult. When you made these adjustments, you perhaps felt disoriented or afraid during these transitions, but you survived and forged ahead into your new environment, just as your baby will be doing. Now that you have completed the transition, have you ever wanted to go back, let's say to the fifth grade, because you missed being there and wanted to repeat the year? Probably not. With each change in the stages of your childhood, you left behind many of the comforting qualities of that life to move ahead into life's next phase, and only a few are willing to go back to their germinal periods of development. Most adults feel better off in their present stage of life than in an earlier one. Looking back on how well you did during these life transitions will give you courage to forge ahead with conviction to do the work of making the changes to create a peaceful womb filled with messenger molecules of unconditional love. The first step in this transition is to build your self-esteem, which will carry you through the upcoming life passages.

Definitions

To work on our self-esteem we need to understand the subject's vernacular, which is confusing. There are several terms used interchangeably. Self-esteem is different from self-acceptance.

Self-acceptance is not being at war with the reality of who we are. It is our inventory of our qualities—both the good and bad. We don't have to like the reality of our inventory contents, but it is important just to accept it. In order to improve ourselves we must know what needs to be changed for the better. We also need to realize that there are parts of us that we cannot change, such as our height, eye color, or race; and there are some changeable qualities, such as our beliefs, habits, and attitudes. The logical step in building self-esteem is to plan to change the less than satisfactory parts of ourselves as much as we can and to accept those that we cannot, the concept so well expressed in the Serenity Prayer. There will be more about this important concept in this chapter when I discuss specific action steps on enhancing self-esteem.

Self-esteem is best defined as the fountainhead of a successful life. It consists of two components: self-confidence, the attitude that you can handle the situation you are facing; and self-worth, the opinion that you deserve happiness, the love of someone, or the promotion at work.

Self-confidence is your opinion about how well you can meet life's challenges. People with self-confidence are ambitious and tend to be creative. They have a sense of being on a journey that they trust will have a great outcome—a life quest. They are supportive and nourish relationships, and they have a sense of adequacy in life. They are not bound by tradition or ritualistic approaches to life's challenges. They are inventive and filled with optimism. They are opportunistic and are not oriented toward safety and security. They are willing to take risks to explore different approaches to solving problems.

Most people go through life not really understanding what makes them happy and waste many years pursuing pleasure, only to find, when the fancied goal is realized, that they are not happy. A popular expression of this concept is that these people are so busy climbing the ladder of success that they don't observe the wall it's leaning against. Happiness is truly a choice not dependent on your surroundings or possessions. It is an internal feeling of being worthy and part or something much larger than yourself. Happiness is having a purpose in life that transcends the intermittent difficulties present in our day-to-day lives. (Again, remember the spiritual optimism of Dr. Frankl and his colleagues in the concentration camp.)

A good gauge of your sense of self-worth is the quality of your romantic relationships. You may think it is a miracle that someone loves you, because you don't value yourself as lovable. If you don't love yourself, then it feels unnatural to have someone love you, and you have difficulty returning their love. In such situations love moves you out of your comfort zone and eventually leads to your subconscious destruction of the relationship. This is true in spite of your opinion about the importance of loving relationships.

On the other hand, loving people with low self-worth is difficult, because they always need reassurance that your love for them is real. Nothing is ever enough to appease their insecurities. They are like a bottomless pit always demanding more and more proof of your love, and you can never make up the deficit.

It is obvious that the most important love relationship you have is with yourself. Without self-love, you can neither give, nor receive love from others. The mistaken concept that one needs to diminish or humble himself in order to love another is a popular misconception that appeals to people with low self-esteem. Simply stated, health is drawn to health. People with high self-esteem choose romantic partners with high self-esteem. They are far more likely to be successful in their romantic endeavors than those who show the self-deprecating love of low self-esteem. This is why it is so important that in every facet of your life you have a deep conviction that your universe is safe and loving, and you are a unique, important part of it. On this conviction hangs your happiness and health, and that of your children and loved ones.

Action Plan for Raising Your Self-esteem

Men and women with good self-esteem don't expect others to fill their dreams, nor do they blame others for their life situations. They accept responsibility for their own predicaments. By just accepting responsibility for your life circumstances, your self-esteem rises.

There is a fine line between this philosophy and the one of taking blame for, or feeling guilty about, all that happens to us. We are not responsible for all the problems we face. Some we can control, while others we cannot, and we have to discern the difference between the two. There are some controllable risks for improving pregnancy outcome like smoking, while other risks are beyond your control and the control of your health care providers.

Accepting responsibility is exhilarating. It empowers you for action. It moves you from being a victim of circumstances to discerning what parts of your life you have control over, and finally to taking action toward improving those you can.

There are two components of self-esteem where action steps are important. They are living authentically and self-acceptance. I will discuss each individually for clarity, but the two areas overlap. Each area will be explored with sentence stemming to find what needs improving, then I will guide you through goal setting and action steps to realize the goal of raising your self-esteem.

Living Authentically

There are times in our lives when we are more true to ourselves, and there are other times when we are afraid to express what we truly are—

an important living part of a friendly universe that was, in its beginning, designed for you. During the times when our behavior is congruent with what we truly are, we are relaxed and experience our genuine selves. We feel adequate to the situation and know that people are responding positively to our authentic self. Other times we try to change ourselves to meet the expectation of the people or the situation at hand. We stuff our genuine self deep into the dark corners of our souls in an attempt to hide our personal truths. During these times our energy level and free flow of ideas and conversation are stifled. This is the distinction between living authentically or not.

None of us can live authentically unless we know what we are. This requires self-acceptance—an accurate inventory of our talents and weaknesses. It does not mean that you have to like every aspect of yourself, just have an accurate assessment. This is the first step in living authentically. We will do some exercises to help develop this inventory that is the foundation for creating a peaceful womb by giving your unborn child unconditional love.

We all have experienced people who gauge how they should act to please us. They constantly want to say what they think we want to hear. They may be pleasant, but they are constantly evaluating the situation and calculating their response. They lack congruence between their talk and actions. I think of them as shallow people with no follow-through. They value your opinion about themselves more than their own. They quickly become boring friends and make unsatisfactory life partners. Like the superstars with professional personas, they are filled with anxiety about being discovered. They don't know how to express their desires in the relationship, because they are afraid of being abandoned.

Remember that you, as a child of God, are important to the universe and have valuable, unique talents. What faults and problem behaviors you may now possess were created by your own actions, which you can undo. (More about this in chapter 14, "Changing Behaviors.")

If you don't feel that you are good enough and must live a life filled with personas and facades, then you have some important work to do. If the person you love is in love with a hallucination that is not authentically you, then you are forced to live with the terror of being discovered. You can never relax and drop the act—a painful existence. But a healthy relationship will always support the authentic you. A loving relationship will always want you to be uniquely you and will encourage you to grow in that unique direction rather than force you to fit a mold, or to suppress part of your personality or one of your talents.

The purpose of the commitment between life partners is to facilitate the spiritual and psychological growth of each other. This requires absolute truth telling, which takes courage. Some fraudulent people tell little lies daily, which is a destructive way to participate in a relationship. Even if the lies are not discovered, the fraud still exists and can never be hidden from the liar or a developing fetus, no matter how good the liar is at suppressing them. The resulting shame is directed inwardly and diminishes self-worth. The fraud destroys a part of self-esteem and is subtly expressed in subversive ways. The eroded self-esteem becomes more destructive to the relationship than the negative effects of truth telling. When one feels and acts this way, what messages is she sending her unborn child?

The key to creating a peaceful womb is to unconditionally love yourself, your life partner, and to feel safe in your universe. The peaceful womb is the responsibility of both you and your life partner, who must make the commitment to join your inner journey of parenting your unborn child. For the sake of the emotional development of your unborn child, you and your life partner must create your own sanctuary of unconditional love. In this relationship you must have the trust of your partner's love to freely express your inner thoughts and feelings. (More about this in chapter 18.)

High self-esteem does not guarantee popularity. In fact, people with it tend to be independent thinkers, more outspoken and open about their feelings. They are self-assertive in a healthy way that may raise envy or even hostility in others. They tend to seek nurturing relationships filled with respect, benevolence, and mutual dignity. They are trustworthy, because they are forthright with their emotions and thoughts and feel comfortable with them.

A good tool to help build your older children's self-esteem is to actively listen to them with good eye contact. Children have a lot to tell us, but have difficulty in putting their thoughts into words. Actively listening to your child and reflecting back what you hear helps him get in touch with his feelings and develops his language skills. These are important skills that will help him later in life. If you are interested in learning more about building your child's self-esteem after his birth, I highly recommend Steve Vannoy's excellent book, *The 10*

Greatest Gifts I Give My Children, which describes tools to teach our children important life skills.[3]

For now you have already read about the importance of parenting your unborn child's emotional development in the section Fetal Parenting. You have established the routine of taking several fetal love breaks a day to create a peaceful womb, which literally shapes the developing child's brain and sets the emotional tone of his neuroendocrine system.

Some people are confused about living authentically, because they have learned during their childhood to deny their feelings. They disown their anger, fear, and pain, and lose all contact with their inner selves. Unfortunately, this inhibits all emotions, including the positive ones like love and joy. Adults who have trouble living authentically usually saw their parents avoiding important issues in their intimate relationships. There was no verbal description of issues, but the walls of the home seem to tell the child's subconscious mind the truths about their parents' feelings. Couples who hide their emotions usually build up so much anger and resentment that when they finally are discussed, the interactions are heated and threatening to children. By this example children learn it is safer to hide their emotions because nothing is resolved. A frightened child, who observes such behavior, develops the attitude: If I value the relationship, I must not rock the boat by discussing distressing issues. More marriages are destroyed by this attitude than by honestly confronting issues with dignity. Learning how to fight fairly is critical to a successful marriage and important to the emotional development of your child, both before and after her birth.

It is essential to let your life partner know what bothers and hurts you. He or she loves you and wants you to be happy, and therefore has an interest in not perpetuating these disturbing problems. It is far wiser to discuss problems when they first come up, than it is to allow them to fester. You must trust the relationship enough to vent your feelings with force and passion.

Remember, you can't hide your feelings from your unborn child. You may choose to try to hide your emotions from your life partner, but your developing child knows exactly what you are feeling. It is far better for you to live authentically, because the active expression of your emotion relieves stress, which changes your brain's neuropeptide message to your unborn child.

Let's get to work on creating an inventory of your authentic living techniques. Get your writing pad, and put at the top of the page, My Personal Inventory on Living Authentically. Then answer each of the following statements with a grade of 1 through 5 with 5 being the best:

I am generally honest with myself about my feelings.

I recognize my feelings and experience them without being compelled to act on them.

I am honest with others about my feelings when the context is appropriate.

I consciously strive to be truthful and accurate in my communication with others—particularly my life partner.

I talk openly and confidently about the things or activities I admire and enjoy.

I talk about being hurt and upset with honesty and integrity when the context is appropriate.

I stick up for myself and honor my own needs and interests.

I share my excitement with others.

When I am wrong, I express it honestly and candidly.

I express to the world the self I feel internally.

Look over the grading of these statements. Do not reproach yourself. Just accept the low marks as a part of you that needs work. Write next to the low marks (say a mark less than 3) a short paragraph describing the problem. Think of possible origins or mechanisms for its development. This will help you receive clarity on the predicament and better self-understanding.

Now turn the page and on the top of each succeeding page complete the following sentence stems:

The hard thing about being honest with myself about my feelings is . . .

The hard thing about being honest with others about my feelings is . . .

If I strove for truth and accuracy in my communications . . .

If I talk openly about the things I love, admire, and enjoy . . .

If I were honest about feeling hurt, angry, or upset . . .

If I were willing to show my excitement . . .

If I were honest about being wrong . . .

Each day, set aside time to review the sentence stems you completed the previous day, and then rewrite them on succeeding pages in your notebook. Becoming authentic will not happen overnight, but this exercise will help you achieve this important goal. It will uncover the problems you have in developing authenticity, and will guide you in mastering this important challenge. Look over your sentence stems and mark the ones that are associated with the low scores in your personal inventory on authentic living. Then set them aside to be worked on later in my book when you learn about setting goals in chapter 19.

As an example, let's suppose that you graded yourself with a 2 on the first statement: I am generally honest with myself about my feelings.

Then in the sentence stems you had the following endings:

The hard thing about being honest with myself about my feelings is . . .

1. I don't feel them.
2. I am not aware of my feelings all the time.
3. I am afraid to be angry, et cetera.

The next day you have the following completions to the same sentence stems:

The hard thing about being honest with myself about my feelings is . . .

1. I might upset people with my anger.
2. My life partner will not love me, et cetera.

Over the next several days as you repeat these exercises, you become more aware that you are afraid to express your anger, because you might lose an important relationship, such as the one with your life partner. Obviously, one of the goals is to learn how to express anger safely. Another goal may be for you and your life partner to learn how to fight fairly in your relationship.

Most of the answers to these inventory questions and sentence stems are personal and should be kept confidential. You may have to explain this to your life partner, because you will not be candid and spontaneous enough if you are concerned that someone might see your answers. This is a good idea in even the most supportive relationships. You don't want to inhibit your responses. A good marriage exercise is for you and your spouse to do the same inventory and sentence stemming, followed by a general discussion, but I still encourage each of you to respect your partner's need to keep the responses confidential. It is good to discuss the general themes discovered in these exercises, and you may ask each other for suggestions and help in goal setting. When doing the action steps leading to your goals, an active partner, who has a sincere interest in your personal development, can help you achieve them.

As a general rule, it is best to keep personal development exercises confidential and share them only with people who are absolutely committed to the goal. You may be surprised at how few people are sincerely interested in your personal development. Be careful here. This is not an area I recommend discussing with social friends. Of course you may recommend my book to them, but keep your goals and your progress private. Well-intentioned friends may be threatened by the unfolding of your self-esteem, and undermine your evolution toward this portentous life realization.

Self-acceptance

If you are worried about the pregnancy, have trouble communicating with your health care provider, are afraid of labor, unwilling to discuss with your work supervisor what changes you need in the workplace, or have a problem with smoking, drinking, or drug use, you must first accept that fact as true before you can change and grow. By accepting what you are and what you are feeling, you will develop a platform from which you can make choices and begin to progress in the direction of your desired change.

If you are not totally pleased with your looks while pregnant, then stand naked in front of a mirror and look carefully at each of your good and bad features. Notice how unique you look. Have you ever wondered why you are so different from everyone else when it would have been so easy for God to make us all look alike? Take an inventory of the features you don't like and decide which ones you can and cannot change. You may be able to change hairstyles while pregnant, but will have to wait for a weight loss until after the baby is born. In fact, it is important to remember that proper weight gain during the pregnancy is important to the health of your unborn child. Too little weight gain is associated with small babies who may have lifelong handicaps from the unadvisable practice of their mothers' trying to stay slim while pregnant.

There may be some things that you can never change like the color or your eyes or your height. The exercise here is not to fight or deny what you see, just categorize the parts you accept and the ones you do not. Then put the unacceptable into the categories of modifiable or not. The process for changing behaviors and attitudes is exactly the same. You first must know the reality of the situation before you can begin the procedure for change.

In my eyes pregnant women become spiritually and physically attractive. There is a serene radiance of fertility and ripeness that is evident in physical appearance—your skin, your eyes, and the way you interact with your partner, as well as with other loved ones. Pregnant women develop a fascinating charm that attracts people's attention. Strangers may approach you with warm words of encouragement or gentle curious comments about your well-being. They view you as attractively vulnerable and naturally want to protect and help you.

Fathers also look and act different. You have a different posture and walk. You stand taller and walk bolder. You possess an air of confidence and pride. You take charge of your infant's mother. You become more protective, and more concerned about their welfare, your future, your job, and the family finances. You are more likely to make purchases, to prepare the home, to think about wills and untoward future circumstances. These changes in appearances and attitudes of enhanced responsibility and protectiveness develop throughout the pregnancy and are known as the nesting reflex.

This primitive instinctual behavior is commonly seen throughout the animal kingdom, and is fun to experience and observe in us humans as well. Relax and enjoy it. Allow your newfound beauty to flow and know that both of you will appeal to the rest of the human race, which will interact uniquely with you.

After you finish this exercise of looking at yourself in the mirror, spend a minute looking deep into your own eyes. Try to look through them into your soul—your very essence. Find your private self, which distinguishes you from all others, and know your uniqueness is good. Get in contact with this essence and allow yourself to feel the goodness within. Accept it as an important component of you and allow your eyes to smile in recognition. Then watch as your entire face evolves into a smile—see it, feel it, and hold that sensation while mentally stating some of the affirmations you have posted around the house.

This is a great way to start the day. I find it a great boost to my self-esteem, because I confirm that I am a valuable child of God with special talents and a specific life mission for the good of the entire universe. That is what I am and why I am here.

Tony Robbins, an author and a personality for motivational TV programs, has coached many highly successful people in America's leading corporations, show business, and professional sports who credit him with turning around their faltering careers. Tony can tell how well his pupils will perform in their business and personal activities by their body posture. As an example he can tell how well the tennis star Andre Agassi will perform by the way he walks into the tennis stadium before a match. He notes the difference in his clients' eye and hand movements when they are doing well and when they are not. He then teaches them how to walk, hold their head and hands like they do after winning an important point or contract. His pupils report that they can change their mental alertness and performance by mimicking the body movements of success. You can learn the same techniques to alter your emotions and alert your brain for maximum performance. If you feel down or afraid, you can build your confidence and optimism using your body.[4]

You and your life partner can teach each other your own movements and postures for each of your moods. Stand facing each other and start telling your partner about the most exciting time in your life when you felt great. A time when you were on top of the world and felt invincible. Have your partner watch your head, eyes, mouth, shoulders, arms, and hands while you relive and describe your feelings during your finest hour.

Linda pointed out that my hands became more active, my eyes widened, and the edges of my mouth curled up while talking about my greatest life achievement. Now, when I awake from a deep sleep to attend a high-risk delivery in the middle of the night, I mentally prepare for being at my best for my patient by just going through these same body motions. I emphasize my hand movements, open my eyes wide, and force a smile; and I feel better. I can come from a deep sleep to a high level of mental alertness and attention in seconds. This skill serves me and my patients well, and it can do the same for you and your unborn child.

During the workday, I exaggerate my body posture and hand movements into one outrageous motion I call a "chest pump." I slap both hands to my chest in a posture like I had just won the Olympic 100-meter race. The "chest pump" is getting a reputation around the hospital, and I am seeing others use it as an expression of celebration. It feels great! Try it.

When you get into the habit of using your body to change your emotions, you are tapping into the rich resource of your psychological potential. You can change your mood and improve your performance. By using proper body movements, you can change from being pessimistic to optimistic. You can switch from feeling helpless to having high self-esteem at times when you need optimal performance. After practicing this skill you can use your body to make you feel the way you want to.

When you start to practice your body-mind connection, exaggerate your movements. You need to go beyond what you may consider appropriate. Go crazy! Become extremely animated when practicing this skill. Be so outrageous with your behavior that you risk possible rejection for being silly. It helps to develop a playful mind-set about this exercise. Make it fun. When you are joyful and relaxed, your mind works at its maximum capacity.

Our minds work like our muscles. In the gym we must do ten to twelve repetitions of the same exercise before we get to the last and most difficult one that gives us the maximum stimulus for growth. Like the exercise enthusiast, you must use extreme effort to train your mind-body connection.

Once these neuromuscular pathways are established through repetitive maximal stimulation, your brain-alerting behaviors become easier. Now when I walk down the hospital hall to attend a high-risk delivery in the middle of the night, I don't have to actually do a "chest pump." All I do is a mental picture of one and I feel my mind preparing for an optimal performance for my patients. This simple technique has made me a much better provider of excellent health care at times when it is difficult for anyone to be at their best. You too can train your body to help your mind be at its best when you are trying to change risky behaviors or prepare for maximal physical effort during labor.

This chapter has offered many different activities and exercises to help you enhance your self-esteem. Some may be easy for you, others more difficult. Again I want to emphasize the importance of not being harsh on yourself. Don't put yourself in an adversarial relationship with the reality of your feelings, habits, or appearance. Do not give yourself the excuse of complaining to your friends about the things you want to change. This tricks your mind into thinking that you are taking action and doing something about it, when actually you are only practicing self-indulgence. The key is to make the commitment to change, set the goal, list measurable action steps, and then start taking small steps one day at a time toward your goal, trusting the power within to help you along.

You will be far more serene about the problems you face by just getting started. It also helps your self-esteem. Do not put yourself in an adversarial relationship with your own opinions and experiences—accept them. Just accept what you are, while remembering that you are a unique and important part of the universe!

Conclusion

Self-esteem determines success. You will do about as well as you think you will in most of life's endeavors. The higher your self-esteem, the more likely you are to be successful. This is why the spiritual philosophy you choose is so important to you, your life partner, and to your children. What you think you are goes right to the core of self-esteem, and that depends on your perception of how important your role is to the world.

Self-acceptance is understanding what you are and not being at war with it. You don't have to like what you are, but before making a change, you must accept it and understand why you are that way. This is the beginning of changing your life and the foundation for building self-esteem. This work requires you to live with the knowledge of both your inner and outer worlds and have the faith that your God-given talents are unique and important to the universe. Using them will bring you love, joy, and prosperity—the perfect environment for birthing and raising children.

12

Setting the Goal to Live Responsibly

We never know how high we are
Till we are called to rise;
And then, if we are true to plan,
Our statures touch the skies.

—*Emily Dickinson*

You are probably asking, "How do I get started on the important work of changing my self-esteem and some unwanted behaviors like the negative chatterbox?" You do it by setting goals and planning action steps that lead you toward achieving these significant life changes. The broad generalities that we all use in setting New Year's resolutions will not work. They may be good ideas, and we may have good intentions; but they are usually too vague, and we lack the necessary follow-through to make them successful; therefore, the majority of resolutions don't last beyond the first two weeks of the year. In chapter 14, "Changing Behaviors," I describe ways to make lasting changes in your behavior, and a part of this important venture is goal setting.

The Power of Setting Goals

There was an interesting study on goal setting among the students of the 1953 graduating class of Princeton University.[1] At graduation, each senior was asked if he (it was an all-male school then) had set goals for his life and if he had written them down. Most of the students said they did not have specific goals. They had some general vague ideals of being happy, wealthy, and having a good marriage. Only 3 percent of the students had taken the time to develop their goals into specific descriptions of what they wanted to achieve during their lives. The ones who had done this and taken the initiative to write them down were more successful in their lives as measured by their total worth twenty years later. In fact, the total worth of the 3 percent of the graduates with goals was more than the collective wealth of the other 97 percent of the class. The point here is that goal setting is powerful, and there is an optimal way of doing it.

First, it is important to write the goal down and make it as specific as possible. Give as much detail as possible and set a time for its achievement. Then write a general paragraph about how you will feel after the goal is finally achieved. Picture yourself at the top of achievement, relax, and let the feeling of success fill you.

Then write about the sensations. Take time with this important step. It presets and brings into action your subconscious mind, and, as we have learned during the sentence-stemming exercises, it is full of knowledge and wisdom. I like to think of our subconscious minds as the part of us connected to the divine, a collective source of wisdom. I try to rely on it more and more in my day-to-day activities, and with practice I have become more facile in its use. You too can develop this wonderful resource.

The next step is to write down the roadblocks in the way of reaching your goal. Again, be specific. Getting your fears down on paper helps you manage them. You then can look them over and develop strategies for controlling them. The next step is to write down the changes that you need to make to overcome these roadblocks. These changes become your action steps, which you will use as milestones to measure the progress toward achieving your goal. Be sure to set dates for each action step and for achieving your final goal. When each action step is accomplished, celebrate by rewarding yourself.

An interesting exercise is to draw a picture of your goal. As an example, when I decided to write this book, I drew a picture of the book's cover and the title page with my name as author. Then I wrote out my goal to have the draft in the hands of an editor by the first of the year. Next, I wrote three pages about how I would feel on the lecture circuit stumping my concepts in the book to large audiences of pregnant families. It was wonderful. The audience was attentive. They even laughed at my jokes. They asked appropriate questions. A few gave personal testimonies to the group about how the book had helped them. It was a powerful fantasy that gave me energy and the initiative to start writing.

I then wrote down all the roadblocks I could think of, like not being able to write well, not having enough money to get the project off the ground, being easily distracted with the other aspects of my career, and receiving peer criticism. Once I had written these objections down on paper, I made some decisions that helped me overcome most of these roadblocks, like hiring an editor, not talking to many of my peers about what I was doing, and making some adjustments in our financial situation with the help of my wife, Linda. Then I made an outline, and set each section of the book up as an action step, and then I was completing my first draft. The fact that I had come this far on such a monumental task gave me the energy to complete it, and I had overcome many of the obstacles that were on that first piece of paper, such as the fear of writing.

Realize that change is hard work, and it is not done overnight. The idea is to set your sights on the horizon and always keep working toward the goal, then set milestones of progress with time frames, so you can measure your accomplishments along the way. Once the action plan is written, do not be afraid to change it as new information comes to you, perhaps from your continued sentence stemming. You may decide that you need more information or help from someone along the way.

Using the fear of expressing anger as an example of a behavior to change, one could set the goal "To freely express my anger to my life partner, without any fear, within the next two months." This is an important goal for both you and your unborn child.

The first action step might be to stop and ask yourself, What do I feel during each conversation with my life partner? and to continue to work on the sentence stems daily for the next three days. That will be one action step, which can easily be completed without help from anyone else. The next action step might be to read about anger using the bibliography in this book, or by going to a library or bookstore to peruse the available books on the subject. This step can be written in your workbook as "To obtain two well-recognized books on anger in the next three days." The follow-up action step is to finish reading them in two weeks.

Another action step might be to start doing some exercises on anger with your life partner the week after completing the book reading, and so on, until you reach your final goal of feeling safe while expressing anger to each other.

Once you learn these skills in the safety of your primary relationship, then you can venture out with your newly found capability into other areas in your life, such as the workplace. If the problem behavior you want to change is anger, be careful in areas of your life where you don't have the same level of support as you do at home.

Pregnancy is a good time to learn and practice these skills, because most families are open to change and are motivated toward improving relationships. Once you have mastered the skills of sentence stemming and match them with the skills described in further chapters of this book, you will have expertise that will serve you well in all areas of your life.

Take Responsibility for Your Attitudes and Behaviors

There is one responsibility that is important in all relationships, including the one with your unborn child. You and only you are responsible for your attitudes and behaviors. No one causes you to be angry or happy, loving or fearful, sexually excited or not interested. Many of us state that people or situations make us angry, loving or sexually aroused. Recognize that this common vernacular for expressing moods is inaccurate. You are responsible for your attitudes and emotions, and they don't control your behavior. You control them both, and they are not linked together. You can be angry without action, or you can take aggressive action without anger. They are separate, and each requires a conscious choice.

This is the essence of self-responsibility and it is the root of personal power over your life circumstances. This stance requires self-esteem and, ironically, it also builds self-esteem. Nothing else in the universe but you has the power of self-responsibility. It is a gift from God that makes us the most godlike creation in the universe. You choose to pursue risky behaviors or not to partake. You decide to be actively involved in the decision-making process during this pregnancy or to be passive. You have the power to change behaviors, to control what you ingest, to practice meditation, to reasonably exercise, and ultimately to improve the outcome of this pregnancy, or you can choose to do otherwise. Realizing your power over situations and making plans to take control are exhilarating. Watching yourself progress through each level of making the change is a strong builder of self-esteem.

Irresponsible living basically means not thinking ahead about the consequences of your present choices and actions. Most irresponsible people are shocked at the consequences of their actions, like the husband who returns home from work and notices that his wife's personal belongings are missing. Later, in counseling, he hears for the first time her accusation that they never talk because he is too tired from work. Being responsible means noticing the reactions of the people and the situations around you, and controlling your impulses. Without this monitoring and control, we always put ourselves in jeopardy. Likewise, people who don't complete a goal-setting sequence are acting irresponsibly and will later wonder why they are not successful.

In changing behavior, we must first be aware of the behavior and its consequences, then realize we are responsible for our own actions and reactions to stimuli that set them up. The next step is to set goals that will adjust the behavior to achieve the desired outcome. This approach has been proven to be much more successful than other quick programs designed to change risky behaviors that are so popular on TV ads. Change is a process with six distinctive stages, and you will be much more likely to succeed in any change in your life if you learn to evaluate where you are on the continuum of change and then institute an action plan to bring you to the next stage of achieving your desired behavior change.

For example, do you know people who live passively and blame others for the problems that exist in their lives? They tend to complain and look for ways to avoid thinking about or acting on the problem. These people are good examples of living irresponsibly. Blaming leaves them as helpless victims and, like children, they are constantly waiting to be rescued.

We all know someone like this, but all of us live irresponsibly in smaller but significant ways. The problem of not actively listening to our spouse or our children is living irresponsibly, and will eventually lead to small wounds being inflicted that over time damage our most important relationships. Each of us needs to at least ask the question about being attentive to loved ones and then decide if that is truly the way we want to live our lives.

Some people are so filled with pain that they are not in touch with the rage that fills them. Many times the rage is misdirected, because they don't understand its source. A good way to deal with anger and rage is to write about them. Do not reject or disown these feelings, but put them on paper where they can be fully expressed and analyzed by you. Remember, these feelings are part of you and you have the right to them. Do not reproach yourself for having them.

The healthy and friendly thing to do for yourself is to get in touch with them. The best way to do this is to relax, using the breathing exercises as described in chapter 19, and then try to bring up the anger or other negative feelings. Remain conscious of the feeling and try to experience it fully while staying passive and relaxed. It will help you to say, or write, "I am now feeling . . . , and I accept it fully." This might make you tense, and if so, go back to concentrating on your breathing and relaxation. This will help you get in touch with these feelings and help you describe them in writing and may even help you discover their origin. Certainly an exercise like this will help relieve emotion and may pay great dividends in reducing self-destructive, risky behaviors.

If you find that you are having trouble accepting this concept and feel resistance to experiencing negative emotions while relaxing, then just accept the resistance. It will begin to resolve once you accept it. The key here is living authentically. Learning about your feelings and how to manage them is different from trying to suppress them. If you accept that you are denying your feelings, then the denial will gradually fade and the emotion will emerge with time, so that you can do this very helpful and healthy exercise. In chapter 17 I describe ways your life partner can help you express anger in nondestructive ways to relieve the tension that can adversely affect your health and that of your unborn child.

You may find the following sentence stems helpful if you have never set life goals and used action steps or if you blame others for your irresponsible living. So get out your workbook and complete the following sentence stems:

If I were to give up blaming my life partner for my unhappiness, I . . .

If I were to accept that I am responsible for the condition of my body, I . . .

If I took responsibility for my feelings . . .

Sometimes when things aren't going well, I make myself helpless by . . .

Sometimes I try to avoid responsibility by blaming . . .

The good thing about making myself helpless is . . .

Sometimes I use self-blame to . . .

If I took more responsibility for the emotional development of my unborn child, I . . .

If I took more responsibility for the success of my relationships . . .

If I took more responsibility for every word I say . . .

If I took responsibility for my feelings . . .

Right now it is clear to me that I . . .

This chapter on setting goals and living responsibly is the first and hardest step in changing behaviors. It takes faith in your ability to make the change happen. Once you are able to recognize the behavior as not being good for you and your unborn child, the next steps along the continuum of changing behaviors are easier. They are described in the following chapter.

13

Assessing Behaviors

A thought which does not result in an action is nothing much,
and an action which does not proceed from a thought is nothing at all.
—George Bernanos

Taking charge of your pregnancy means assessing your behaviors and determining which are healthful and good, and which may be detrimental. This chapter will help you with this process that is important in starting you along the path of changing unwanted behaviors.

Guilt

In part 1, I presented the value of our so-called negative emotions. There is one exception. Guilt has no value. It is a detrimental negative emotion that we need to eliminate.

Guilt is associated with judgments, and most of us think that if an important person knew what we had done, they would criticize and possibly reject us. I certainly grew up thinking that if my parents knew some of the things I did, they would not love me. I even bought into the myth that I had to protect my parents from all the bad that happened because their knowing might upset them. Now I know that my mother wants to know what is going on in my life, and what I am thinking. There is nothing I can do to break her love of me. She accepts me with all my faults. I am sure if my father were still alive, it would be the same with him. Guilt should not be part of an important relationship like one between children and parents, or between life partners. Let go of old guilt now. It is a gift to both you and your unborn child.

In my practice, most families with a bad pregnancy outcome suffer from guilt. They invariably ask me about what they did, or did not do, to cause the bad outcome. I try, with compassion, to dispel the myths that are at the center of their beliefs and behaviors, but sometimes after I have given them the best clinical information for the bad outcome, they still reproach themselves with guilt.

There was one exceptional patient who was as clean of contrition as any I have consoled. She was a well-educated, forty-two-year-old woman who had spent twenty years of her professional life in special education, helping children with birth defects. She dealt with many children born with Down's syndrome in her classes, and she knew that at her age she was at risk for having such a child. She was offered, but declined, prenatal amniocentesis, which would have given her the option to abort a Down's fetus.

When she arrived in the hospital to deliver her infant, she told me she had a repetitive dream of her baby looking like a child with Down's syndrome. And he did. This woman was well informed about the care such children require, and she had intentionally declined the diagnostic test that would have given her the option to avoid her situation. She was self-assured and had no guilt about her pregnancy resulting in a mentally retarded child. She was an exceptional woman.

In most situations where a child with a birth defect is born, or a pregnancy ends with a premature birth, there is a great deal of guilt and second-guessing about what should have been done, or what was done that adversely affected the pregnancy outcome. This woman had a much broader perspective on the problem. She was knowledgeable about the relationship between her age and Down's syndrome, she had carefully evaluated her options, accepted the risks, and was comfortable with the consequences. She is an example from which we can all learn.

When people feel guilty, they diminish their self-worth and try to justify or hide their behavior. This only makes the situation worse. With a lower self-worth we are more likely to regress into the behaviors that cause guilt, and we enter into a spiral of repetitive negative behaviors that are hard to correct unless we eliminate the guilt.

So how should we respond to a guilty feeling? Use it as a trigger to examine and correct the behavior. This is the only way to eliminate guilt from our lives.

Building a Platform of Self-acceptance

Preserving your integrity and self-esteem has huge consequences for your health and happiness and for the mental health of your unborn child, as you saw in earlier chapters. It's important to realize your own value system as distinct and separate from someone else's.

We all start developing values by assimilating them from people we respect. We first accept our parents' values, but during the adolescent years we begin to test their importance while developing our own. This time of exploration is an important stage, and it may be years before we recognize our values as guiding principles for decision making.

To assume responsibility for your behaviors and their consequences, you must become aware of your feelings, and learn how to safely express them. Remember, you have every right to your feelings and thoughts, but they don't control your behavior. You choose to act on them. Recognizing this distinction gives you power over unwanted behaviors.

Children get mixed messages when parents don't share the same values. For example, their mother may be good at saving money and caring for possessions like clothes, while their dad may neglect possessions and not be as frugal. We learn by observing and mimicking people we respect. You and your life partner may have different values, so take the necessary steps to mesh them as quickly as possible. How can you instill your value system into your children without first fully recognizing your own and accepting that of your partner?

Start with these sentence stems to determine how you would function if you were more independent in your own thinking.

If I express my feelings freely . . .

I act on my feelings when . . .

If I were willing to see what I see and know what I know . . .

Remember that what we think and do are all expressions of ourselves, but none of them defines us. We all have attributes that we would like to discard and others we would like to develop.

To help solidify your platform of self-acceptance, try the following sentence stems:

It is not easy for me to be self-accepting when I . . .

It is not easy for me to admit . . .

One of the emotions I have trouble accepting is . . .

One of my actions I have trouble accepting is . . .

One of the things about my body I have trouble accepting is . . .

If I were accepting of my body, . . .

If I were accepting of the bad things I have done . . .

If I were accepting of the good things I have done . . .

If I were accepting of my feelings . . .

If I were honest about my wants and needs . . .

The scary thing about being self-accepting is . . .

As I relax, breathe deeply, and allow myself to experience self-acceptance . . .

These sentence stems will show you why self-acceptance is so important to making positive changes in your life. If you refuse to accept your feelings and behaviors, then how will you be able to make the changes required to correct risky behaviors? You cannot forgive yourself for behaviors you have not recognized as being part of yourself.

Now, in your notebook, list five or six facts about yourself that you would like to change during this pregnancy. Remember that these negative aspects of you do not define you. They are a few negative attributes among your many positive ones. You are only trying to get them out on paper as a focal point to work on them. Accepting them does not mean you like them.

Now complete these sentence stems:

As I accept the changes in my behavior that I need to make during this pregnancy, I . . .

The hard thing about accepting ———— is . . .

If I were to accept ————— completely . . .

I am becoming aware . . .

As I accept the changes this pregnancy brings to my life, I . . .

A good finishing-up assignment to this rather difficult and possibly self-deprecating exercise is to discover how much you really like yourself. Let go and really acknowledge the good person you are with the following sentence stem:

If I were to admit secretly how much I like myself . . .

Some people reward themselves for denigrating themselves. They think that others will reject them if they value themselves too much, and then they will have no excuses for complaining about their spouse, their boss, their parents; or, people will expect much more of them, expecting them to control unwanted behaviors, which they would rather not.

Quite the contrary is true! People are much more attracted to someone with a strong sense of what they are—and perhaps what they are not—along with the knowledge that they are in charge of who they are and how they act.

Managing Guilt

Just like any behavior, guilt can be managed. Please answer the following questions either to yourself or in your notebook: When feeling guilty, do you seek to understand the guilt producing behaviors by considering the options you had at the time you started the behavior? Do you generalize your negative feelings of guilt to other areas in your life, or do you keep them tightly associated with the specific behavior? Finally, do you try to learn from the regretted actions, or do you just keep repeating them and remain stuck in the same old behavior patterns?

Some people have much higher expectations for their own behaviors than for others'. Do you assess your behavior the same way you would someone else's? For example, are you more likely to give someone an excuse for being late to an appointment, while admonishing yourself for being just as tardy? Are you more critical of behaviors in yourself that you accept in others? If you answer these questions affirmatively, you are probably responding to guilt.

Guilt can either be a strong motivator to change behavior, or it can paralyze you. This depends on how it affects your self-concept. When guilt diminishes self-worth, it paralyzes your ability to stop repetitive behavior patterns in a self-fulfilling prophecy. Some people use generalizations as alibis for not taking action to correct obviously negative behavior, such as smoking. They will say that they have smoked all their lives, and they know many people who have smoked and lived longer than they want to. They would rather remain in the familiar misery that provides a weird type of coziness, not expecting much from themselves.

Such passivity is a cop-out. If they did away with the self-reproach, they might progress and grow into new psychological territory, which could be frightening. They feel that happiness requires more psychological risk than they are willing to assume. They choose to remain in those familiar miserable places that have provided comfort for them. This self-destructive behavior cannot be corrected as long as they keep telling themselves how bad they are.

A good way to break out of the comfort zone of repeated unhealthy behaviors is to go back in your past to embrace and love the person you were when the behaviors started. This may take you back before your teenage years, well into your childhood.

You've already acknowledged that what you are doing is not good. Now analyze it from the viewpoint of how you were trying to care for yourself. What was the context of the situation when the behavior first occurred? Did you think it was the correct thing to do at the time? Possibly it was the only way you knew how to handle the situation, and it might have been the best choice at the time.

Your actions are always related to your efforts to avoid pain and fear, in other words, to nurture yourself, a worthwhile activity. Sometimes it encompasses self-destructive behavior. Allow yourself understanding and compassion for what you did at that time. This does not mean denying the existence of risky behavior, nor the fact that it is bad for you now. Just accept that you did it while trying to nurture yourself in some misguided way, which can be corrected now with some work. You are now in a different psychological place and view the past risky behavior as unwanted.

A good start to changing a habit is to practice the mental imagery of yourself manifesting the desired behavior, while doing the progressive meditative exercises described in the last chapter of this section. Once you have a clear picture of yourself doing the new behavior, mentally place yourself in situations you now recognize as challenging. See yourself overcoming the challenge, such as refusing a cigarette in a smoke-filled room while enjoying the company of friends who use nicotine.

But be gentle with yourself. You might want to start with a far less challenging situation in the real world than the situation you may have visualized. After all, if you can accomplish something that difficult in your head, succeeding at something less daunting will be just as exhilarating. For example, try eating a meal and instead of lighting up a cigarette afterward, take a walk. This is a powerful way to change behavior. Most of us underestimate our abilities to make changes for our good health.

Mental imagery is powerful. An interesting study of college basketball players at a major university with an excellent sports psychology program offers just one example. Psychologists divided the team into two groups. The first group practiced free throws for thirty minutes in the usual way of going out on the court and shooting the ball through the basket. The second group only did the mental exercise of making free throws in pressure-filled game situations when the points were critical to winning the contest.

When the two groups' performances were compared in actual game situations, the group that practiced with mental imagery alone outperformed the group who had practiced using the classic practice approach. Now most teams who practice sports psychology combine the two methods. And it will work for you, too.

When you start to feel guilty for an action—or nonaction—first forgive yourself for the behavior. Recognize that the behavior is not you. It is just part of all the different expressions that make up your overall person. Certainly there are many other actions that constitute good behavior. You, with all of your God-given talents, are capable of choosing behavior to relieve guilt. Be kind and give yourself the accolades you deserve when doing the right thing. Remember, you are unique in the universe and have many talents to use in changing your unwanted behavior. God is forgiving and does not want you to waste your talents on self-destructive behaviors that produce guilt.

Disapproving Family and Friends

My wife, Linda, can send me a certain look from across a room, and I will immediately get the message that I am behaving in some way that displeases her. My sensitivity to her expressions developed from knowing her so well and loving her so much.

The disapproval of the people closest to us is responsible for a lot of the guilt we experience. You may not consider a behavior as being detrimental, such as having an occasional glass of wine while pregnant, but a close loved one may rebuke you, and that may elicit guilty feelings.

Take a minute to listen to your inner voice and use your own standards to judge the behavior. Sometimes our feelings of guilt are a smoke screen for feelings of resentment that we would rather not admit. How dare you disapprove of a behavior I find acceptable? It's very easy at this point to get into a never-ending loop of finding fault with each other, snapping shut, cutting off discussion, and harboring ill feelings. Instead, get in touch with the resentment and anger and deal with it.

Your body image during pregnancy is a common area that provokes anger and resentment. The majority of women I have counseled have a mental concept of their ideal appearance, which does not match the way they look when pregnant. This may lead to eating habits that they know are not good for the pregnancy but that support their ideal appearance. This may also provoke guilt.

Some expectant mothers accept their pregnant body image, and I surely hope that is true for you. If your life partner or other loved ones comment negatively, you should feel anger, and now is the time to recognize it and make the commitment to express it honestly.

The following sentence stems may help deal with resentment and anger expressed as guilt:

If I weren't feeling guilty, I . . .

If I were willing to be honest about my anger, I . . .

If what I am feeling is not really guilt, I . . .

A loving relationship should allow free expression of anger. We all feel anger and its full expression should not threaten our loving relationships. Fighting is actually healthy. The key here is to fight fairly, and learn how to let go of grudges. A good fight allows you to express your feelings with passion, and that will give you a sense of relief.

You may have decided that you don't want to assume the awesome responsibility of the pregnancy outcome, and some well-meaning relatives may constantly remind you of this neglected responsibility. I think that's unlikely if you have come this far in this book, but if this should pertain to you, here comes another burden. It is far healthier and wiser to own up to the discrepancy between you and the well-meaning relative, and to tell them how you resent their being a behavior sheriff. Tell them you have made a conscious choice, why you feel that way, and to please back off.

You'll not only feel better but this act will be a benefit to your developing fetus. Remember, he experiences your emotions—and the sense of well-being from taking charge of your life is inestimable.

14

Changing Behaviors

Use what language you will,
you can never say anything but what you are.
—*Ralph Waldo Emerson*

Have you noticed that the world is in constant change, and that it seems to accelerate with each decade? Although we recognize that change is inevitable, none of us much likes it. Some fear it and diligently try to avoid it; but by accepting change as part of life and by concentrating solely on your own response to it—for this is the only aspect of change you can control—you can greatly improve your health, happiness, and the success of your quests.

Pregnancy is an outstanding opportunity to change behaviors for several important reasons. You have a renewed consciousness of responsibility and connectedness to all that is important, which naturally brings you and your life partner into evaluating your beliefs, values, and behaviors.

Pregnancy represents a big change for both you and your family for the rest of your lives. As the trailblazer for your pregnancy quest, I want to guide you through the process for making lasting changes for the good of your health and that of your developing child. All this responsibility can be terribly frightening, but because you are fully committed to making your child's birth and life the best, you already understand, "If this is going to be, it is up to me." Try these sentence stems:

I feel defensive when . . .

Now that I am pregnant I . . .

If I could I would . . .

The purpose of this chapter is to provide you with the best available methods for controlling behaviors. You have already read the information on spiritual awareness, the power of prayer, and the importance of high self-esteem, which are all necessary for controlling risky behaviors. You've learned the importance of self-acceptance and forgiving yourself for past behaviors. Now it is time to apply specific techniques to change behaviors.

Most popular cessation programs for risky behaviors are intensive workshops that give you information about the risks of behaviors and then some techniques on controlling them. Their success rate at best is about 25 percent, with the rest lapsing back into their old ways. The main reason for these paltry results is the simple fact that we are not all at the same stage in the process of change. Those who are ready for the action stage as described by Dr. Allen Prochaska in his book *Changing for Good* will succeed.[1] The others are still operating in one of the three earlier stages of change.

I like Prochaska's work and find it to have the greatest efficacy among a multitude of programs. Let's get to work now starting your own change process by discovering which stage you are currently in and then how to progress to the next while continuously enhancing your self-esteem.

Dr. Allen Prochaska, a clinical psychologist, started his career by studying all the different disciplines of psychiatry, and his work led to the astounding conclusion that no psychiatric discipline was clearly superior to another, and that most people can make changes without the help of therapy.

He then became fascinated by the process of change and discovered some basic principals involved in changing all behaviors. It does not make much difference if an individual is in therapy with a mental health professional or not. In fact, the majority of people who make significant changes in their lives never seek professional help. Thirty million people have quit smoking on their own, which is twenty times greater than the number who have quit with the aid of a treatment program.

If you want to use a mental health professional to help with changing behavior, make sure that you find one who understands the process of change. Dr. Prochaska believes that mental health professionals actually function as coaches, while the work of change (including that which occurs in psychotherapy) is solely up to the individual.

Most people think that change occurs abruptly and simply requires willpower. Dr. Prochaska has shown through his study of thousands of people that change follows a predictable course, and the key to successfully changing your behaviors is not willpower alone, but the application of the correct strategy at the appropriate stage in the change process. Each of us needs to know where we are along the change continuum, and then apply the correct procedure to progress to the next stage.

There are six stages of change, starting with precontemplation and ending with termination of the unwanted behavior. There are nine processes to use to progress through each stage of the change continuum.

Moving from Precontemplation to Contemplation: Why Change?

Precontemplation is the first of the six stages. People in this stage don't think they have a problem, although others perceive its existence. Precontemplators don't want change. In fact, they view the people around them as the problem and think they are the ones who need to change.

The first step is to understand that change is up to you and not the people around you. You can begin the process of change simply by accepting that you can do it. It doesn't have to be right now, but it will eventually happen if you progress along the complete continuum of stages. A loved one who is willing to work on your behalf could help to educate and motivate you from precontemplation into the stage of contemplation.

Contemplators acknowledge that they have a problem and desire new behaviors. They are just not ready to do it. They seek the final piece of information that will make the change easier and guarantee them success. This seeking activity is actually outright procrastination—usually from the fear of failure. But you have learned and practiced techniques to overcome fear. So, no excuses. When contemplators begin to focus on solutions rather than the problem and begin to think more about the future than the past, they become filled with anticipation and activity, which helps them prepare for the next stage—preparation.

Return to the sentence stems you did at the beginning of the chapter and list the changes you would like to make now in your life. For each one, grade your response from 1 to 5 for the following four statements. The grading scale is 1 = never, and 5 = repeatedly. The assertions are:

1. I look for information related to my problem behavior.
2. I think about information from articles and books on how to overcome my problem.
3. I read about people who have successfully changed.
4. I recall information that people have given me about the benefits of changing my problem.

According to Dr. Prochaska, precontemplators score less than 10, and a score greater than 10 indicates that you are beyond precontemplation and into contemplation, or one of the higher stages of change.

Giving Up Guilt

What did you discover in the last chapter about the feelings of guilt that you may be dragging around? Remember, don't deny or ignore them—just explore them. This is probably the hardest and most important step to take, because denying responsibility for the guilt-inducing behavior is one way to avoid punishing ourselves for behaviors we know are not beneficial.

Your life partner can help raise your level of consciousness and provide useful information about problem behaviors. She can also help with improving the environment by not smoking around you or starting an exercise program with you, or helping you select a better diet and set up a schedule of times when you both can practice relaxation techniques and mental imagery. Some people have the unfortunate misconception that it is necessary for precontemplators to hit bottom before trying to help them. This is inefficient, painful, and risky.

If someone you love had life-threatening cancer, would you wait for undeniable signs of the cancer before trying to help them? Of course not, and the same is true for behaviors. The longer people wait to change behaviors, the more difficult it is to change. Some precontemplators give up on themselves because they are demoralized. They give in to their problems and feel life has passed them by. They are resigned to unhealthy behaviors.

You can help yourself move from precontemplation to contemplation by taking responsibility for your behavior and by forgiving yourself for starting it in the first place. Remember that it served your needs when you started it. It was a loving thing to do, as maligned and misguided as that may seem at this time in your life. At the time it served your best interest, but now you are in a different place emotionally and psychologically. Change is inevitable, and it is time to accept it and move on.

If another person has been affected adversely by your behavior, make amends now. This relieves the guilt that recycles the unwanted behavior, and confessing it improves your self-esteem. This takes courage, but I have found that most people I have hurt are forgiving when I confess my feelings of guilt and ask their forgiveness. They typically have a broader and more philosophical view of the situation from a different perspective. When you learn to better understand and forgive yourself, your self-concept and behavior improve naturally. Guilt is really a form of self-indulgence that none of us can afford.

Don't assign virtue to your feelings of guilt and remorse. Harshness about yourself is nothing to boast about. It leaves you passive and powerless. Suffering does not inspire change. It traps you in the cycle of negative behavior and guilt. Suffering is one of the easiest of all human activities, while creating your own happiness is one of the hardest, because it calls for emancipation from guilt.

I know you are concerned about your pregnancy because you are reading this book. You've probably found some of the ideas and exercises easy to follow. Others may not have been so easy. Some pregnant women don't want to take responsibility for the pregnancy. They may not have the stamina or willingness to do all the exercises I am suggesting. They may not accept the spiritual philosophy or the power of prayer. They may not be able to control their fears with the exercises I suggest. If you fall back into old habits of blaming yourself for your lack of commitment, you will just pile on more guilt trying to relieve it.

Please, relax. Think through the reasons for poor follow-through, if that's been your case, and remember it does not define you. It does not mean that you are an uncaring mother. Remember the exercises that help explore the reasons for behavior. Maybe you're not very excited about this pregnancy. After all, it is a heavy responsibility, and will forever change your life. Again, sentence stemming may help you explore your own feelings about this important area. They will certainly clarify your values.

You may be worried about the effects this pregnancy will have on your career, your marriage, your financial future, and your leisure time. These are all legitimate concerns, but the difference is that you now understand how to work through these problems to make decisions about balancing your life goals.

To give up guilt, you need to explore beyond your feelings into the realm of your expectations and values. We may set lofty goals, an admirable endeavor, but unrealistic goals lead to failure and guilt when they are not consummated.

Do not give up your goal, but be gentle in evaluating your progress toward it. If you become discouraged about an important goal, break up the process of achieving it into smaller action steps, and reward yourself upon reaching each of them. Remember to control your internal chatterbox. A positive reinforcement is more effective than a negative admonition in changing behavior patterns. Using positive affirmations stated in the present tense speeds your progress toward your laudable goals. A few examples may be the following statements.

I now let go of my past mistakes, which frees me of my guilty feelings.

I am a unique part of the universe.

I am making progress toward my goal of doing all the exercises presented in Loving Your Unborn Child.

What are some additional specific positive affirmations you want for yourself? Please add them to your notebook now.

Getting the Help You Want

As a general rule, I don't tell people about my goals. Not everyone is supportive of my self-development. I don't want to hear their negative or questioning comments, because I want to remain focused and optimistic.

Before telling anyone about my goals, I try to evaluate how supportive they are toward my attaining them. I am more likely to tell friends about goals to stop negative behaviors than I am to tell them about goals of accomplishments. They are more likely to be critical of the latter, but they will remind me when I stray from the narrow path of correcting negative behaviors. This is human nature. Your challenge is to learn how to use it to your advantage, and to stay focused forward on what is important to you.

Loved ones who want to support your personal development will be helpful. If they are not, then they may be part of the problem. For example, a couple who smokes may want to keep each other smoking to relieve their guilt for not having the strength to quit. When one member of the couple recognizes that anyone smoking in the home is a detriment to the health of their developing fetus and will lead to more respiratory illnesses in their newly born child, there is a strong and valid incentive for stopping anyone from smoking in the house. This is an excellent opportunity for both members of the couple to work as a team to eliminate the risky behavior in their environment. Each can act as a mentor for the other.

Change from Risky to Healthy Behaviors

A word about risky behaviors. Most readers think of smoking, drinking alcohol, or using drugs, but I am also talking about more subtle behaviors such as not exercising or eating improperly, not communicating clearly with your medical team, or not doing the fetal love work of meditation with mental imagery during the fetal love breaks that are important to the health of your fetus. These minor but still risky behaviors are not talked about frequently, but you now know they are all-important keys to successfully parenting your unborn child. The same skills presented here to control risky behaviors can also be used to reinforce positive behavior changes. Not doing a positive behavior can be just as detrimental to the pregnancy and to your self-esteem as doing a destructive one. People who want to change behaviors should consider making several changes at once. The process is the same and replacing a negative behavior like smoking or drinking alcohol with new positive ones such as exercise and meditation facilitates progress along the change continuum and increases the probability of success.

Getting Beyond Precontemplation

Was your score low on the assessment of precontemplation? If so, you should spend time with the two processes used in moving from precontemplation to contemplation—consciousness-raising and social liberalization. The first involves the use of information that makes it easier to choose wise alternatives to the unwanted behavior. The second recognizes that more information about risky behaviors is available, and society is offering more conducive environments for positive change, such as nonsmoking areas in public places.

Helpful relationships are important in many aspects of our lives, and making behavioral changes is no exception. You need to select someone as your change partner who is committed to your personal growth and change. This may or may not be your life partner, but whoever it is can help by making accurate assessments of your unwanted behavior. Your life partner may be afraid to be too critical or you may not accept his criticisms. If so, choose someone else to be your change partner—a dedicated person who will give you information to raise your consciousness, and help you see yourself as others do.

We are all defensive about unwanted behaviors, but our defenses rarely fool others, especially loved ones close to us. Just by asking a loved one to help with changing unwanted behaviors is an important step in breaking down defenses.

Change partners must be patient, because they may want you to change too rapidly, and they may push you into action before you are ready. Their primary role in the precontemplation stage is to be the voice of reality for those who are powerless to change without assistance. This is a difficult task that takes tact, but a change partner should know how to motivate you by pushing the right buttons. This does not mean nagging, but it also means not being an enabler who softens the blow of the negative behaviors by covering up their consequences.

Sentence stemming will help identify your defense mechanisms. Here are a few sentence stems to get you started. Share your answers with your change partner to give him or her added insights to help you in the best possible way.

I feel defensive when . . .

Doing ———— makes me feel defensive because . . .

When you do ⎯⎯⎯⎯⎯, I feel defensive because . . .

When I feel defensive, I . . .

Also evaluate how socially liberal your group of friends is by looking at who is for or against your risky behavior. Do they represent your best interest? What will that person lose or gain if you change the behavior? Those who will be hurt by the positive change in behavior are not the ones who will support you through the change process and are not good change partners.

Consciousness-Raising and Emotional Arousal— Keys to Preparation

Raising your level of consciousness about unwanted behaviors is a good way to move from contemplation to the stage of preparation. Start by asking questions of experts and people you trust. Most people, when they become ill, go see a health care professional, or when their car breaks down, depend on a mechanic's expertise. No one will try to fix their car or cure a serious illness without asking questions and getting advice from experts, yet most of us think we can change behaviors without seeking help. This is absurd. You need to begin to ask questions and evaluate your behaviors.

Pull out your notebook right now or write your answers to these sentence stems to help raise your consciousness and to do a functional analysis on your exercise behavior, as an example.

I neglect safe exercise because . . .

I don't exercise because I . . .

When I don't do these exercises, I . . .

I justify not doing this exercises by . . .

If you want to analyze another behavior, you can substitute any behavior for the word *exercise* in the above sentence stems.

The Process of Self-reevaluation

An important change process is self-reevaluation, which is the cognitive and emotional appraisal of your behaviors. Review your responses to the previous sentence stems presented in this chapter to gain insight into the emotional aspects of your unwanted behaviors. Ask yourself, or your change partner, if the unwanted behavior is in conflict with your value system. Be honestly critical. This is the time to be courageous and look carefully at the inventory of what you don't like in your life and what you want to change to attain your desired improvements.

Pregnant families usually are willing to look at their health behaviors and make lifestyle adjustments that provide a positive impact on their unborn child's health. Make a list of both the positive and negative aspects of the behaviors you want to change. Include the consequences of the change to you, your unborn child, and others. Then try to imagine and list the reactions that you and the others will have when the behaviors change. Think about how you can explain your risky behavior during this pregnancy to your child when she or he is old enough to understand.

Try the following sentence stems to explore this important area of self-improvement in perinatal health:

What I dislike about [unwanted behavior] is . . .

What I like about [unwanted behavior] is . . .

If my unborn baby knew I was doing [unwanted behavior], he . . .

When I change my [unwanted behavior] . . .

When I change my [unwanted behavior], [name of person] will . . .

The reality of prematurity in the United States is staggering. More babies are born early in the United States than in most of the other industrialized nations. Most of these infants survive after the painful and expensive experience of neonatal intensive care. A significant percentage suffer lifelong handicaps like an IQ less than 70, blindness, deafness, or other central nervous system disorders such as cerebral palsy or hydrocephalus. Fifteen to 20 percent of prematurely born children will have respiratory conditions that require hospital readmissions.

There is presently case law that supports a child's right to claim damages against his mother's employers for prenatal injuries related to her work site. Soon the day will come when a child will sue his or her mother for participating in risky behaviors during her pregnancy. Use your imagi-

nation and think about the adequacy of your defense for not fully participating in all healthful behaviors during this pregnancy. Could you win
the case? What defense could possibly justify your unhealthy behavior?

Preparation

Preparation, the next stage, is the cornerstone of a successful self-
change effort, and it must precede action. In fact, action without
preparation is likely to fail. During the preparation stage you are planning how to make the change. This is the time to focus on the future
and self-reevaluation. You may fear failure during this stage. Mental
imagery skills are helpful in producing mental pictures of how your life
will be with the desired behavior change. Use these skills to help you
progress through the preparation stage. Develop mental pictures of
yourself enjoying your new behaviors. Remember to turn of your negative chatterbox by replacing it with affirmations.

A major part of preparation is planning. You need to set a date for
when to make the change. More important, you need to think about
all the situations that will tempt you to revert back to old behaviors.
Discuss with your change partner how you will counter these temptations so he or she can help you even better in implementing your plan.
Sentence stemming will help you recognize the situations that are
likely to set you back when you move into the action stage.

When I start exercising, I will . . .

. . . is likely to make me not want to exercise.

When I don't feel like exercising, I will . . .

Now add some sentence stems that may be even more appropriate
for you. Of course you can substitute any behavior for the word *exercise*.

Going into Action

People often equate the action stage with behavior changes, but you
can see why these preliminary stages are so important. Dr. Prochaska's
data suggest that the self-changers who don't do adequate work in contemplation and preparation are likely to relapse to old behaviors.

Most of us know how to start this stage, but we lose our commitment soon after initiating our good intentions. There are several important processes that help us stay the course in changing our behaviors.

Countering

Countering is a very useful change process during the action stage. It basically is the substitution of a positive behavior for the undesirable one. If you remove troubling behaviors without replacing them with positive ones, the risk of relapse is high. Exercise is the most useful countering behavior for many negative behaviors, and we'll look at it in detail in chapter 19. You will learn to transfer your urges for the risky behavior into cues for positive behavior like exercise or relaxation, prayer, and meditation, which also are good countering techniques.

To be successful at countering, you need to change your thinking patterns from negative condemning ones to affirmations in the present tense. Work on self-talk. Remember to keep it positive and in the present tense. If you have not yet developed this important tool for self-help, go back and review "Controlling Your Chatterbox" in chapter 10. Do not neglect the exercise and practice. Like all new skills, they take work and time before you become proficient at them. Be gentle with yourself. You have already started making many necessary changes.

Self-responsibility

Sometimes you may subvert your efforts to maintain positive behaviors because of fear of self-responsibility and social isolation. If you obtain your lofty goal, you may no longer be popular is how the myth goes. I frequently hear "It's lonely at the top," but I firmly believe that to forgo your positive goals and deflate your self-esteem in the name of popularity is leading you into a new kind of loneliness, a loneliness where you are surrounded by friends more interested in protecting their self-images than in helping you grow and develop your personal potential.

Would you want your children to obtain the same goal you are striving for, or would you rather they be fearful or question the virtues and positive attributes that you now desire? We all want the best for our children, but at the same time we may be hesitant to own the same distinction for ourselves.

To own and take pleasure in what is best within ourselves is not to become boastful and arrogant, but to have the satisfying sense of accomplishing an important goal. On the other hand, we must not diminish ourselves by settling for less than what we can achieve, or by lying about who we are. Goal setting requires personal integrity and self-understanding.

It takes courage to be honest about our assets and liabilities. Here are some sentence stems to help you in this area. You know the routine, so here goes:

If I have trouble accepting any of my assets, it might be . . .

When I feel defensive about positive circumstances . . .

The scary thing about admitting pride in myself for my accomplishments is . . .

If I were willing to admit to things I feel pride about . . .

The emotional reward of accepting your attributes will be immediate and positive. As with most benefits, there is the risk of your acceptance of your talents alienating people with low self-esteem. This will put new pressure on relationships, and you may have to assess their value in face of your personal growth. This will cause some turmoil in your life for a while, but you will soon attract people with better self-esteem who will facilitate your personal growth. Once you start down this road of personal and spiritual development, it is difficult to stop. Health is attracted to health, and your growth will gain its own momentum.

Your life belongs to you, so please follow what is natural and pleasing and accept the consequences. This is your natural-born right, which is protected by our nation's constitution and supported by our most admired institutions, including the church. In spite of society's acceptance of this concept, many people feel that they don't deserve these inalienable rights. They have been taught that their primary role is to serve, first their parents, then their spouse, and finally their children. These responsibilities are put before their own happiness.

This unfortunate psychological set-up is more common among women than men. A man is admired when he fights for what he wants, but a woman fighting for personal growth may be criticized for being selfish or overly assertive. Fortunately, American society is in the process of reevaluating the disparity between the gender roles. I know that both men and women can be ambitious, kind, and nurturing all at the same time. One personality trait is not diminished by the development of another. We are multifaceted and can have all these qualities.

Sometimes women have to be told that their lives belong to them, and they have the same rights as men to pursue their interests and talents to the same extent. No one who really loves you will want to stifle your self-development. People who want you to serve them don't truly love you. They want to keep you in the mold of their expectations, which will prohibit your personal development. Your most important asset for personal growth is your life partner, and anyone who truly loves you will facilitate the development of your unique ideal. This is the epitome of love, the willingness to work on behalf of another so they can be uniquely themselves.

Okay, end of sermon. But it felt good to say it to you, because I know how good you'll feel as you do this work.

Assertiveness: Defending Your Rights

People confuse assertiveness with aggressiveness or anger, but there is an important yet subtle difference. Assertiveness is declaring your rights that are held equally by everyone. You, like everyone, have the right to be heard, to make mistakes, to change your mind, to judge your own thoughts and feelings while resisting those of others, and to set limits while asking others to respect them.

Aggressive behavior makes the statement, "I count but you don't," and passive nonassertive behavior makes the statement, "You count but I don't." Aggressive people usually hurt others, while assertiveness accomplishes goals not at the expense of others. It gives others the opportunity to understand your objectives and asks them to join with you, which greatly increases your chances of changing behaviors.

Maintenance: The Art of Sustaining Change

You may have heard a smoker say, "Quitting is easy. I quit smoking twenty times a day." What is difficult is sustaining the desired behavior changes over a lifetime, because, as everyone knows, slipping back into old behaviors is easy and happens frequently.

Maintenance is not a static process of willpower over temptation. It is a time of learning, activity, and growth. The two important fundamental elements of maintenance are long-term effort and a revised lifestyle. We already looked at the process of "countering." Here's the other important technique.

Environmental Control: Using Cues Properly

Environmental control involves changing the situations that lead to the unwanted behavior. This is different from countering, which involves changing your response to tempting situations. The three basic methods of environmental control are: avoidance, use of cues, and reminders.

Avoidance is the key to controlling environment, because it helps eliminate temptation. Many people mistakenly rely on willpower alone to resist temptation, when avoidance is more helpful. It simply means staying away from the environments that tempt you into the unwanted behaviors.

Obviously you can't go through the rest of your life avoiding temptation. Eventually you will face an environment filled with temptations. The proper use of cues helps you face the tempting environments; the key is to practice using them when you feel safe. Imagine yourself in a triggering environment such as your workplace under the stress of a deadline. Visualize yourself taking a deep breath, relaxing, and successfully performing the desired behavior of taking a fetal love break. Positive mental visualization is an important psychological tool to be used by anyone interested in maximizing their performance under stress. Professional athletes have been using it for the last decade and now businesspeople are using it to rehearse success in stressful situations. I use the method while preparing for a difficult delivery of an extremely premature infant. You can develop the same skills to prepare you for problematic situations—they're laid out in the last chapter.

For reminders, set up a schedule and mark your calendar for regular participation in countering behaviors like exercise, relaxation, and meditation. Keep your schedule in an easily seen place like the door of the refrigerator or in your daily organizer. Finally, check off the accomplished task when you complete it—one of life's little but extremely powerful pleasures.

Using Rewards: Treats for Good Behaviors

Reward your efforts for positive changes. Many think they should not be doing the risky behavior in the first place, therefore they don't deserve the rewards for the change. It is a mistake to punish yourself for past mistakes. This deceptive thinking leads to relapses, and the way to avoid them is to use rewards liberally for the small successes you make along the change continuum. Here are three techniques for rewarding yourself—covert management, contracting, and shaping up.

Covert Management

Covert management is the self-talk we use when confronting a cue. Remember to relax first and then coach yourself through the situation with words of encouragement. Use the same words you received as a child from a supportive parent or coach. Even if you did not have positive parents, imagine what it would be like to receive good words of encouragement and congratulations from them at this time.

Remember, your unconscious mind can't distinguish reality from what you imagine, and using positive self-talk while confronting a strong cue trains your subconscious mind to resist your unwanted behavior while enhancing your self-esteem. Negative self-talk sets us up for future failures when we repeat the same negative self-talk messages.

The word *motion* is an important part of the word *emotion*. Our activities and emotions are tightly linked to each other. We can change our emotions by going through the motions as described in the section on self-acceptance in chapter 11. Our emotions affect how we perform in so many ways, including our physical movements. When we watch athletes, we observe how they can get in a groove of high performance they call the "White Zone." They prepare themselves for optimal performance by going through a ritual of body movements that help them build confidence that they will perform optimally under stress.

Stay away from using covert punishment. It only increases emotional distress and decreases self-esteem. Getting angry at yourself for something you did or did not do is not helpful. The berating usually happens after the fact, when you have already enjoyed the rewards of the act and it is too late for any negative self-talk to be effective. It is important to be gentle on yourself and to remember that changing behaviors is a process with ups and downs. You will succeed at making the necessary changes in spite of slips into old undesirable behavior patterns. You do this by remaining positive in self-talk and by developing the skills learned throughout this book.

Contracting

Contracting with yourself for the desired behavior change is an effective covert mechanism for behavior control. It uses the reward mechanism and continues the process of building self-esteem. For example, when you hit the ideal weight gain of twenty-five to forty pounds during pregnancy, contract to reward yourself after the baby is born with a one-year membership to a gym to help you lose the weight gained. You will learn techniques for contracting with your life partner in the chapter, "Learning to Fight Fairly." You may want to contract with your change partner to do mutual work on changing each others' behaviors and lives. You will both benefit.

Shaping Up

Shaping up is an important process. Change is gradual and takes time. You overcome unwanted behaviors gradually by shaping the change you want in your behavior. The process involves several steps toward your goal. At each step, reward yourself. Make the first step small and easy, and even though you don't think you deserve it, reward yourself. Be easy on yourself and make the shaping-up process joyful and playful by being curious and adventuresome with your rewards. Try something new like you did as a child. Your state of mind is important to you and your loved ones, and is most important to your unborn child. Unknowingly we influence people more by our state of mind than by what we say to them.

A second benefit to shaping up is that when you slip (and you probably will), this will help to avoid falling all the way back to the beginning. Well-practiced, well-rewarded earlier steps are good ways of keeping the small slips from becoming complete relapses.

Slips and Relapses—Learning by the Recycling Processes

There are three internal challenges often associated with relapses. One is the overconfidence that you can handle any environment or temptation. The second is the daily temptation you face. Typically you get overconfident and think you have the problem beat and one little slip will not be detrimental. But, alas, the statistics show this is wrong. Slips do lead to relapses.

The third challenge is for you to eliminate self-blame if you should have a slip or relapse. If you continue to blame yourself for failures, the entire change effort often backfires. Most people think self-blame controls behavior, when it actually demoralizes and stymies your growth. Self-blame does not belong in your thinking. Counter it with positive self-talk and by changing your state of mind using the body-mind connection described later in this section.

Research data show that people who slip or relapse into old unwanted behaviors, but were eventually successful in making the behavior change, don't quit on themselves. They simply forgive their mistakes and start over at an earlier stage of the change continuum—perhaps at contemplation or preparation—and try again. Most successful changers view the process as a spiral of successes and relapses until finally the desired change sticks. They use the periods of slips and relapses as learning opportunities to reevaluate the processes that failed them. The most common mistake made is not budgeting enough time for the effort of making changes in behavior.

A relapse is not a failure! If it happens to you, do not make the mistake of thinking that the reason for the relapse is lack of willpower. When relapses occur, it is best to rely on countering behaviors that you have learned, and to call on your change partner to help you evaluate what went wrong and correct the problem by trying something new. Again, I strongly urge you to make this a playful process. Be adventuresome and creative. Don't give up. Use your mind, body, and change partner to improve on the skills and change processes about which you have already learned.

Most relapses occur during times of psychological stress and social pressures. Go back to your action plan and devise new ways of coping with the situations that led to the relapse through relaxation, meditation, exercise, and countering techniques. But one word of caution—don't become a chronic contemplator. Step out and keep taking the risk of going into action after careful evaluation.

If you believe you will make a change, it will happen! You will learn through the slips and relapse experiences how to make the changes you want. Success is an attitude, and starting anything new requires a leap of faith. Count on your passion and attitude! Review the chapters on your beliefs and the power of prayer. Your belief that the universe is safe and you are an important part of it can help you work through slips and relapses. You'll get there!

15

Good Communication Builds Strong Bonds: What You Can Do Now

Nurture is above nature.

—Proverbs

The work of bonding with your unborn child does not come automatically or naturally. It requires your willingness to work on your thoughts and emotions. Not doing the work of communicating with your unborn child is a risky behavior that, tragically, most parents and health care providers neglect. We're all aware of the risks of drinking and smoking, but American medicine does not emphasize the benefits of the behaviors presented in this book. They are not as well studied as drinking and smoking, but the clinical evidence indicates they are equally, if not more, beneficial to your unborn child. Most of my colleagues are more interested in treating diseases than in bolstering health and development. This is why the work presented in the next five chapters is so important. To communicate well with your unborn child, you will need to know how to recognize and safely express your emotions to your life partner, support group, and health care providers.

It is amazing to me how closely mothers are emotionally linked to their unborn children. At no other time in our lives do we so clearly communicate our thoughts and feelings as mothers do to their developing children in utero. What a marvelous system to have in place during this important time of psychological and emotional development. All the problems of verbal communication that we adults so frequently encounter are completely eliminated. Don't miss this opportunity to give unconditional love to your developing child. Remember, fetal love work lasts a lifetime.

Wouldn't it be wonderful to communicate clearly all of our thoughts to each other all the time? Or would it? Think about it. There would be no way to hide feelings and thoughts from loved ones. We may expect our life partners to read our minds and to know intuitively what we need and want because they love us, but that is impossible. We must make our wishes and thoughts known through clear communication, and it is a good thing that we have some control over which thoughts are communicated, because not all of them are worthy or appropriate.

Your developing baby is in the position of receiving all of your thoughts and emotions, whether they are worthy or appropriate or not. You cannot hide or modify them. This presents you with a big responsibility. You probably want to send her only loving messages of reassurance. However, she shares all of your emotions, both the good and bad ones. Don't worry about this. You have read how to give your unborn child positive fetal love messages by taking fetal love breaks. You don't have to think bright and happy thoughts twenty-four hours a day. Just be sure that you take the time to relax and use mental imagery to send powerful positive messages richly filled with love neurotransmitters.

The occasional doubt, anxiety, or negative emotion will not permanently damage your unborn child. Fear is part of pregnancy. What is harmful is how consistently you are anxious and how you feel about your pregnancy. If you are constantly fearful and view yourself in a hostile environment, then your baby will have the same sentiments.

The most important way to counter this potentially harmful effect is to practice the exercises presented throughout this book that help you control negative emotions such as anger and fear. You have learned how to develop a positive attitude about your environment, self-esteem, and how to communicate your belief in self-importance to your unborn baby and to the universe. Remember, *you are* the universe to your fetus.

You have learned that the universe is a friendly place. You have read about World War II prisoners who found positive meaning in suffering and were able to transcend the atrocities of the Nazi concentration camps. You have learned about the power of prayer, setting goals, and self-talk. These are all tools that will help you control fear and anxiety. The World War II prisoners used them. If they overcame their horrible conditions to develop spiritual optimism, certainly with persistence and training you can also overcome the adverse conditions you face.

Your input into the psychological development of your unborn child cannot be duplicated at any other time in his life. The feelings of being loved and wanted that are perceived from the edge of his developing consciousness are important gifts with major impacts that last a lifetime. He shares your view of the world. You are the conduit of your unborn baby's emotional experience. This is why it is so important to have strong faith and a good understanding of your importance to the universe and to grasp the personal power of prayer and positive self-talk. You can do this by following the simple exercises in this book. Please make the commitment to do this important work.

You are probably now thinking about what type of emotional stress you are experiencing, and how much harm you have done to your unborn child. Dennis Stott in the early 1970s concluded that short-term, fairly intense stress during pregnancy did not adversely affect the fetus.[1] He found that long-term personal stresses that were either continuous or unpredictable caused the most damage to the fetus, because they released the largest amounts of stress neuropeptides. This result is similar to the study done with monkeys exposed to stress using the three degrees of food supply. The positive neurotransmitters of love and acceptance neutralize the adverse effects of these negative experiences.

Ignoring your unborn child is like leaving him alone in his room for nine months. He has emotional needs just like the rest of us. Pregnant families should give their unborn children as much psychological countenance as they can muster during this critical period of neurological development.

Unborn babies kick when they are aggravated or anxious. When you feel your baby kicking, you can console him by rubbing your abdomen while singing and talking to him. Abdominal rubbing is a universal behavior of pregnant women in most of the world's cultures.

Try this experiment. Ask your baby's father to place his head close to your uterus and yell loudly. This will create a kicking reaction in a twenty-eight-week-old fetus. Then place earphones on your abdomen, and play your favorite soothing music loud enough so your infant can hear it. You will experience a quieting response in your fetus. Be sure to play the type of music I wrote about earlier. Hard rock or rap music is not relaxing to your unborn child.

Are you excited about your power to nurture your unborn child? The love you give him now will return in abundance during the many years you will be parenting him. Your relationship with him now is less filled with distracting stimuli, and you have more control over his sensory input now than you will have after his birth. Let me, your trailblazer, guide you in your quest to make the best of this incredible opportunity. Read on to learn the skills you will need to give these important gifts to your unborn child.

16

*N*urturing Your Unborn Child Through Communication with Your Life Partner

From hearing comes wisdom; from speaking repentance.

—*Proverbs*

When I see the face of a contented newborn, I am often reminded of my father's expression while boarding his sailboat during our last visit together before his death. My father had several heart attacks before he died, and he was a man of great courage and faith. He and I wrote and talked about the end of his life, and how he had a sense of completion and a readiness to meet his beloved savior. Like most challenges in his life, he looked at his impending death as a great adventure.

His death was not unlike, but certainly much grander than, the adventures he and I shared sailing. Each time we sailed from the harbor there was uncertainty, and after we reached our destination, we shared the pleasing satisfaction of successfully navigating our small boat over a large span of troubled, and on occasion dangerous, waters.

Because of my own religious beliefs, I know in my heart that when my father had completed his final great adventure and spiritually reached his eternal resting place, his face was like I saw it during our last visit together on his sailboat. And to describe his joy when he saw his savior, I first have to describe my own feelings when I was reunited with my wife, Linda, after a stressful period.

After a twenty-four-hour call in the hospital, I rushed to an important date with Linda, who was waiting for me in New York City. We had tickets to see Radio City Music Hall's Christmas Pageant. It was a greatly anticipated event for us both, having bought the tickets months before the show date. I was tired from my interrupted sleep, and after making checkout rounds, I rushed to the train station to catch the 11:00 A.M. train from Philadelphia to Penn Station in New York City.

During my rounds, the train ride, and the taxi ride, my anxiety increased with each slight delay. I was stressed and anxious from the fear of not meeting Linda before show time. This was an experience we both had looked forward to sharing for years.

As I approached the theater's entrance, I heard Linda's voice over the din of street noise calling my name. At first I could not find her in the gathered crowd, then I saw her running to greet me with a warm embrace and a fragrant kiss. I had made it! The sense of relief and accomplishment was palpable in my heart, and when I looked into her excited face I felt blessed, satisfied, and safe.

My reunion with Linda is the only life experience I can use to relate to what I have seen many times in the delivery room, and during my last visit with my father on his sailboat. It is an insignificant comparison to the response my father had meeting his savior, and to the many contented smiles I have seen on newborns when they first see their mother's face after their travail of labor and birth.

These three experiences are examples of many common life experiences, varying in degrees of importance. Obviously my arriving on time to meet my wife for an exciting event does not compare to my father's last visit, but I believe there is nothing during our lifetime, except a possible near-death experience, that can compare to the newborn infant's experience of first seeing his mother's face. I likened the newborn's experience to the spiritual meeting of my father and his savior. After all, for the past nine months, the newborn's mother has been his sole provider and protector. You provide all that your unborn child needs to grow and develop from a single cell into the universe's most revered creation. As God is to me, you are your baby's ultimate provider and protector.

I cannot describe God, nor do I fully understand Him. I only know that He is there and loves me. This gives me the comfort and courage to step out boldly during my life. At times it is difficult to believe and understand why God loves us when we feel so insignificant and undeserving in the big scheme of the universe, which I believe is a friendly and loving place in which to live and die. It helps to think about my relationship with God by using my knowledge of an unborn child's relationship to his mother. Like my relationship with God, your unborn child is not aware how he is intimately connected to you, his loving mother, but medical science is learning that he is conscious of your presence in mysterious and powerful ways. I believe it is impossible for the fetus to understand how this communication occurs; yet the two of you do communicate in a personal and powerful way.

My relationship with God helps me be more productive and, I believe, a better person. Your emotional relationship with your unborn child helps him became a well-adjusted child and eventually a better adult. Now, during pregnancy, is the time when the neuropathways are developing that will determine how he will react to the life adventures that lay before him. If you view your environment as hostile and are angry or have other intense negative emotions toward your life partner, your job, or to life in general, there is an excellent chance your child will too.

Love and communication are common themes that run through my book. I have written about your special place in the universe, and how to use prayer to communicate with God and build self-esteem. You have read about the skills to change how you think about yourself, your fears, your unborn child, and God. Now is the time to develop your consciousness about your emotions and to learn how to express them in honest, open ways that are safe for you, your life partner, and your unborn child. In this chapter you will learn to communicate with the most important person in your life—your life partner. In chapter 19, you will learn how to communicate better with your unborn child and prepare for his most important life event—birth. You already know the mechanisms and importance of communicating with him.

The Secrets of a Successful Intimate Relationship

Our communication with loved ones usually emanates from our emotions about them; therefore, it tends to be more expressive than cerebral. This is different from the way we talk with friends and colleagues at work. Communication in a loving relationship is more frank and honest, and emotions are likely to flow freely. This is the way it should be, but at times, when emotions are high, the words we use hurt the ones we love and the relationship that is so important to our happiness. Ideally we communicate with loved ones in ways that foster our love for one another, but sometimes this is not the way it works out. When it doesn't, it hurts all of us, including our unborn children.

To facilitate healthy communication among your loved ones, you will need the following skills:

1. The safe and effective expression of your feelings
2. The development of good listening skills
3. The skill to fight fairly for change

Each is important to your relationship with your life partner, and to your children, born and unborn. Children obviously thrive when their parents have a healthy relationship. It has also been shown that committed couples with good interpersonal skills have fewer illnesses and live longer than people living alone or who experience chronic tension with their life partner. We are designed to be in a loving relationship.

I view my marriage as a workshop for my spiritual and psychological growth. My first priority in my relationship with my wife, Linda, is to help her develop into the person she wants to be. This does not mean the person I want her to be, but the spiritual, emotional, and intellectual person she desires to be. I am most proud when she is excited about what she is achieving in her life, because I know that all she does comes from the nurturing love I give her. In return I receive the same love and nurturing from her. Having experienced this, I now understand what philosophers mean when they write, "To receive love you must first give it away."

Improving Communication Between You and Your Life Partner

A healthy ritual for you and your life partner to develop is to set a time for communication each day. This can be structured around a meal, or some other repeated protocol in your daily lives, like putting children to bed. At first, the structure may seem strained and your conversation will lack spontaneity, but with time and practice the habit will become easier and spontaneity will return. This is a time to nurture your relationship, and the work you are doing is an act of love for yourself, your partner, and your unborn child—the significant people in your life. This is essential, and it takes discipline, but once the habit is formed, the rewards are well worth the effort.

Dr. Virginia Satir calls this time of confiding in each other the Daily Temperature Reading.[1] It is a time for intimate clear communication about the big and little things in life that are so important to the success of our relationships. When you can open up to someone without any masks or pretenses, it invigorates the relationship, builds your self-esteem and that of your partner, and sends a very positive love message to your unborn child.

The Daily Temperature Reading is divided into five sections, and takes couples about fifteen to thirty minutes to complete. At first, it may take longer, because the discussions in each section may be prolonged, but with practice the time commitment decreases while the benefits increase.

Step one of the Daily Temperature Reading is called Appreciations. Each person discloses something they value about the other. It can be a simple act of kindness, the way the person looks, or a major accomplishment. We all enjoy adulation. It is good for our self-esteem to hear the one we love compliment us. Some people are their own worst critics, but who is better able to tell you what is good about yourself than the one closest to you?

New Information is step two. This alleviates many of the problems that may arise from assumptions in your relationship. Assumptions can be dangerous, as they are often wrong, and factual information is the simple cure.

The third step, Puzzles, is an interesting exercise. Each of you asks a question. It can be simple and mundane or provocative and possibly inflammatory. Don't be afraid to ask difficult questions. They are the crucible of intimacy. This is an opportunity to test the relationship's response to intimate inquiries. Without the courage to ask provocative questions, one is left with only assumptions about important issues that often lead to misunderstandings and resentments. Remember to dare to be intimate. This may be painful in the short term, but will serve you well in the unfolding of your relationship. You both must learn to trust the relationship enough to risk anger.

I think the most courageous action we can take is to confess our thoughts and actions in the face of possibly destroying a loving relationship. It is far better to face the fear, using the skills you have learned, and confront current relationship issues than to allow them to remain unchallenged. They often reappear in the future in subtle, well-disguised ways that make solving them much more difficult. The lack of courage to discuss current relationship problems damages relationships instead of protecting them.

The fourth step is Complaints and Request for Change. The complaints should not be blaming or judgmental. They are simple statements about what will improve the relationship from your point of view. Keep the complaints specific about behaviors that are bothering you. Then give suggestions on ways to change the behavior or situation. Do not use this as an opportunity to build a list of don'ts. Keep the complaints and requests current. Again, the purpose is to provide information to prevent misunderstandings. Revisiting old problems without relevance to the present situation will not foster relationship development.

The Wishes, Hopes, and Dreams section is the final step, and a time to reflect on what you want from your partner, and from life. This will let each of you learn about the plans and interests of the other. You may discover similar likes and goals. Talking about and visualizing these goals will help you take the next step toward actualizing them.

Taking a Daily Temperature Reading is a great time to practice communication skills. Once you make the commitment to do this exercise daily for several weeks, you know there will be ample opportunity for you to express your concerns. It also gives you the opportunity to practice active listening.

The golden rule of good communication is to first understand before attempting to be understood. Most of us, when discussing an important issue, worry so much about what we are going to say, that we don't concentrate on what is being said. We listen with the intent to judge and rebut rather than to understand with empathy what is being said. The best way to actively listen is to repeat back to the speaker in your own words what you heard him or her say. That assures both of you that the message is understood. Again, this will help correct assumptions, which are damaging to the relationship. When you don't fully understand what is being said, ask for clarification. Never be embarrassed by asking for explanations. Such questions demonstrate empathy. Try to feel what your partner is feeling. Reflect back the emotions and try to understand his or her viewpoint.

After fully understanding and expressing empathy for your partner's message, you can make your statement. When a person is assured that her message has been understood, she is more open to hearing and understanding what her partner is saying. When talking, it is important to be congruent, which means speaking directly while expressing your emotions. Keep your statements as "I" statements rather than "you" statements, which tend to infer blame and assumptions. I feel . . . I think . . . It hurts me when . . . are much less threatening and more likely to convey an accurate message than sentences that start with "you." Remember, this exercise is about helping your relationship. Always think about what is best for the relationship—especially when you are angry.

Believe me, this is not an easy task. When Linda and I have arguments, I can feel the emotional intensity build within me. It is not easy for me to put our relationship before my point of view when I feel Linda is attacking me; but when I sense my emotions rising, I call upon the relaxation techniques I practice each morning. This may not work for you at first, but with practice the skill increases and the response can be immediate in the middle of a heated argument.

A neat suggestion made by Dr. Lori Gordon is for couples to sit facing one another with their knees touching and holding hands while doing the Daily Temperature Reading. When you are touching and in close contact with your partner, you are more likely to work through pain and anger successfully and avoid misunderstandings. This is important, because when you get upset or angry you will want to pull back and look away. This is natural, but make the commitment to keep in physical contact with each other while doing this exercise. The tendency to pull away is an excellent physical cue that you are upset and should start working on relaxing. Remember, your goal is to exchange information and improve the relationship, and the best way to do this is in a low-key fashion. This is not the time to express anger. Anger needs to be released, but there are other more constructive exercises for managing this important emotion.

Assumptions: The Land Mines in the Relationship Field

Assumptions are relationship land mines. Some couples have the unfortunate misconception that if their life partner really loved them, they would know how to please them. This is not true. No one has the ability to read our minds. It is up to each of us to express clearly to our life partners what we need and how they can please us. Likewise, don't expect your partner to understand how you feel unless you are willing to express your feelings. As scary as it may be to express how you are feeling to the most important person in your life, the only way to find truth in your relationship is to face the fear and do it anyway.

Most people venture into relationships with assumptions and expectations. Some of the common ones are:

Loving me means . . . not interrupting me when I'm talking, thinking, or working.

Loving me means . . . knowing what I want and what I feel.

Loving me means . . . not trying to control me.

Loving me means . . . agreeing.

Loving me means . . . needing me.

These relationship land mines are discussed in detail in Dr. Lori Gordon's book *Love Knots*.[2] Now try to discover some of your own land minds by completing the following sentence stems.

Loving me means . . .

If you love me . . .

Loving you is . . .

If I could change you . . .

If you could change me . . .

Anger

There are times when we are angry with our partner and we do not want to be rational. We only want to resolve the conflict by mustering might. We use intimidation, ultimatums, and physical fervor to get what we want. Winning is all-important, and we often make the mistake of acting on our anger rather than just expressing it. Or, we take the opposite approach of suppressing the rage, which is just as harmful. We need to learn to express the anger without harming the relationship. When we suppress anger, we turn it inward, which can affect our health. A pregnant mother cannot hide her anger from her fetus. Her emotions are too intimately connected to him through the neuroendocrine system.

Dr. George Bach, the author of *Intimate Enemy*,[3] believes that the way to deal with anger is to confront it. He has developed several exercises to help people express anger without destroying their relationships. This hard work requires the commitment of both people in the intimate relationship. You work together as a couple to manage anger.

Dr. Bach's exercises allow the angry person to fully express rage with the permission of the listener and the understanding that you both will return to love and methods of resolving the issues that prompted the anger. It is far easier on your life partner when she or he has given permission for you to express anger; otherwise your explosion of rage will be seen as an attack that either elicits a counterattack or withdrawal—both of which are detrimental to your relationship. When permission is granted, you can both work on relieving the anger, and the listener can feel like a helper rather than the object of an ambush.

Dr. Bach describes two rituals for expressing anger. One is the Vesuvius. It allows your anger to erupt like a volcano while your partner respectfully witnesses its expression. He does not participate in the expression, nor should he defend himself or support your anger. He remains passive.

The rules of the Vesuvius exercise are:

1. The angry partner must ask permission to do a Vesuvius.
2. Both parties agree on a time limit, usually two minutes.
3. If permission is not granted, then the two parties make a date for the Vesuvius ritual within the next twenty-four hours. Remember, men may need some time to be alone and think.
4. When it is time for the Vesuvius, the angry member is allowed to express the full extent of anger. This is the time to let it all out and not worry about what is being said or how it is being interpreted. Just let it go and put some energy behind it. The listener's job is to sit passively and keep time.

This technique, which my wife and I use, helps relationships in several ways. It trains fight-phobic people to express their anger, and it helps hot-tempered people manage rage. The listener learns to hear the anger without taking responsibility for the speaker's emotions. Finally, the ritual clears the air and calms the angry person, which allows love and rationality to follow the outburst. These are important lessons for a healthy intimate relationship.

Anger is part of the package of emotions given to each of us and it is usually grouped with other negative emotions, such as fear. I have already discussed fear and explained that all of our emotions, both the negative and positive ones, serve us. Anger and fear certainly protect us from dangers in our environment, and give us energy to either combat the dangers or run from them. You have learned to face fear in part 2.

We are each in control of our own emotions. How we react to what happens in our environment is a choice. No matter what happens, we can choose to be frightened or angry, or to respond with love and compassion. Remember, our emotions are expressed through our neuroendocrine system, and their physical expression helps elimination. It keeps the molecules of emotion flowing so they will dissipate in the body. Damage to our health occurs when the negative emotions don't have an outlet for expression. If the permission process delays the expression of anger, then the angry member is left to her own imagination to discover nondestructive ways for expressing it. This is her responsibility, not her partner's.

A good nondestructive vent for rage is vigorous physical exercise that involves the large muscle groups, such as running. Another is to beat a punching bag or a pillow with your fists or plastic bat.

The first time I witnessed "bat work" I was horrified. I was in a group of health professionals learning about psychodrama, and I did not understand "bat work." The individual doing "bat work" was a gentle, quiet man, whom I thought I knew fairly well; but I did not recognize him during the ten minutes he intensely beat a pillow with a plastic bat. Afterward I talked with him about the experience. He told me it made him feel great. He felt relief after doing it. I could tell this was true from his eyes. He was at peace, while also exhilarated, after the experience. I thought this was strange, and I did not trust it.

Later it was my turn to do "bat work." I was angry, but embarrassed to express rage so wantonly in front of a group of my respected colleagues. I was forced to participate by the class leader and encouraged by the group, and as I expended energy beating the pillow, more and more anger welled up, which brought greater intensity to my physical exertion. I was amazed at the depth of my feelings and how much physical energy I poured into my "bat work."

As unique as this experience was, the most remarkable part of it was the feeling of peace and joy I had after beating the pillow till I was exhausted. There is definitely a physical and psychological benefit to expressing anger in a nondestructive way. There were no feelings of guilt, and I had no worries about repercussions from my rage. I felt relief. Now I can get the same relief from the Vesuvius exercise. What a gift to myself and to my relationship. With these techniques and watching Linda effectively use the energy she gets from her anger, I have made progress in recognizing when I am angry and have learned how to more effectively use the energy anger creates.

As the passive listener to a Vesuvius, you may need to psychologically distance yourself, if the rage is against you. It is best not to get caught up in the emotion, but rather to listen to the message. You may learn some important things that can benefit your relationship. Try to see the situation from your partner's perspective. At the end of the time limit, if your partner wants more time, granting it is up to you. You may want permission for your own Vesuvius, if you are responding with anger, and you then reverse roles. After venting anger you both are better able to work constructively on the issues behind the hostility.

The Haircut is the second ritual for expressing anger. It contains the same rules as the Vesuvius. The difference is that you are blaming your partner for the anger. It is not intended to change behavior. It is only an expression of a gripe.

Another rule that is helpful when dealing with anger is the Belt Line. This is a limit set by each of you that the other must respect. Some behaviors are just too inflammatory to be part of either exercise and are labeled "below the belt line." Two common belt-line issues set by intimate couples are name-calling and dragging past grievances into the present. Each couple establishes their own belt lines, and it is up to them to police and respect the rule.

After any anger ritual, the listener can call the belt-line rule saying that the raging partner went too far. Each belt line should be recorded for future review and modification. Some people name only a few issues as being below the belt line, which allows the partner to run all over them, while others have too many, which usually means they are too sensitive. Both of these extremes are self-esteem issues, and their roots should be explored using the sentence stems presented in this book's section on self-esteem.

After a Haircut, if the listener feels that he is in the "doghouse" for some transgression, he can ask for a "doghouse release," which is not a promise to change a behavior (this comes later with the use of a different technique), but rather a pleasurable gift for the angry partner. This can be a back rub, a present, or participation in an activity enjoyed by the aggrieved partner.

Creating Changes in Your Life Partner's Behavior

The process for changing behaviors in an intimate relationship is called a Fair Fight for Change, from the book *The Inner Enemy* by George Bach.[4] Actually, it is a negotiation process on behalf of a better relationship, rather than a fight against your partner. It is important for the emotional aspects of the behavior to be dealt with, using the above techniques, before entering this negotiation process. For the process to work, both partners need to share the goal of improving their relationship. It is not a barter system for divvying up responsibilities. Each request for change is handled individually and weighed on its own merits.

The process begins when one partner asks permission to engage in a Fair Fight for Change. Then, using the rules of sitting while facing each other and not interrupting one another, the process begins with a period of reflection by the one asking for the change. It is important to compose the complaint using "I" sentences and to state it simply and directly. Logic is the key in this system. Do not use the Fair Fight for Change as a method of attacking your partner. We have already discussed how to vent anger.

The second step is for the listener to give feedback so there is no misunderstanding about the complaint. If the feedback is not clear or incomplete, then the complaint is restated; and this continues until it is clearly understood. It is important that you both understand the complaint before proceeding.

Once both parties are confident that the complaint has been received and understood, there is a second period of quiet reflection, after which the request for change in behavior is presented. It should be specific as to what you want, and within the listener's capacity to give. Be specific and do not overload. Change is made in small steps taken one at a time. Remember, the purpose of the request for change is to build value for the relationship. The feedback procedure is then repeated until both partners are confident that the request is understood.

Then the presenter should ask if the listener is willing to contract for the requested change. This should be followed by a kiss and thanks to the listener for working on understanding the complaint and request for change. The show of affection should be offered even if the listener is unwilling to go further with the process. This is followed by another period of quiet reflection.

During this quiet period for contemplation, the burdens of clear communication and doing what is best for the relationship are shifted from the presenter to the listener. He or she needs to ponder the question, "Can I live with the requested change?" Time-out may be needed for the listener to collect his/her thoughts. The listener's integrity is on the line. It is far worse to make a commitment that will later be broken just for the sake of keeping a short-term peace. It is far better for the relationship to deny a request at this juncture than to contract for a change and default later on. Negotiation and compromises are the principal components of this process, and the ability of you and your life partner to use these components constructively is important to the future health of your relationship and that of your unborn child.

Once the listener is ready to give a response and feedback, the rules about repeating what is stated by each continues, but the basic process changes from one partner being just a presenter or listener to both partners shifting roles during the negotiation process. During this period of negotiation there is the risk of a breakdown in the rules for communication. If tempers flare, you can always shift back to a Haircut or Vesuvius, then return to the negotiation. After the change in behavior has been agreed upon, the couple then sets a date for reevaluation.

This is a great skill to learn and will help build intimacy in your relationship. I suggest you start with small problems and requests for change to learn the skills and procedures, but the process can be used for making big changes in the relationship as well.

There are some issues in every relationship that are not up for negotiation and compromises. These are called "walking issues," which are so important to our personal identity that they are not negotiable. If one such issue should come up in a Fair Fight for Change, then it should clearly be declared as a walking issue, which means it is not open to negotiation. You should never assume that your partner shares your important values, and the only way to discover what values are or are not shared is to discuss them using this constructive format.

My wife, Linda, and I have used the process to make big decisions like moving to a new city for my career. This required her to sell her business and to move from her family for the first time in her life. After many Haircuts and Fair Fights for Change, we learned a great deal about what we each valued. It is an excellent exercise in clarifying values, which is the foundation of the decision making discussed later.

We asked some close friends of ours to help in the Fair Fight for Change process. They were a couple committed to helping our relationship and had learned these skills. They helped clarify our communication, and during the reflection time, they helped each of us consider alternatives and issues that neither Linda nor I had thought about. It took us several weeks to get through all the feelings and to develop a clear understanding of what we each wanted from the move and career change. Our Fair Fight for Change ended with a written contract of changes in behavior, most of which were my responsibility before we made the move. Now Linda states that the move was one of the best things she has ever done, and our relationship is certainly stronger for going through the difficult negotiation period. We have more respect for and a clearer understanding of each other's values.

These processes of mutual self-disclosure are important for building emotional intimacy and they require trust and acceptance. Each partner needs the right to express him/herself without the fear of moral condemnation or attack, either verbally or physically. This is the foundation for a family and a healthy environment for your developing fetus.

The Benefits to Your Developing Fetus of a Sound Intimate Relationship

There is more information being presented in the obstetrical literature about the important, but still poorly understood, connection between a mother's emotional condition and the chances of her going into preterm labor. Women who feel they have no control over their life situation and are constantly afraid or depressed are more likely to either have a miscarriage or go into preterm labor. Some health care providers now use clinical markers that are secreted from the base of our brains that are associated with high anxiety, anger, depression; and the presence of these negative neuropeptides in a pregnant woman's blood indicates she is unlikely to reach term.

Now you have read about many skills to reduce the secretion of these negative neurotransmitters. You have the basis for properly parenting your unborn child to health and happiness for the rest of his life.

$\mathcal{L}$earning to Fight Fairly

Most conversations are monologues delivered in the presence of a witness.

—*Margaret Miller*

It may seem odd to bring up fighting, which is associated with anger and resentment, but a healthy relationship is essential to parenting your unborn child, building self-esteem, and changing behaviors. Expressing your honest emotions, both positive and negative ones, is the cornerstone of a healthy intimate relationship, and this requires clear, regular communication and an accurate self-concept. It is more difficult to have a devoted emotional relationship than it is to have a physically intimate one, and the former is more important, to you and to your family's health.

Many people with careers think their acceptance by and value in society are based on their career performance. I certainly have that conception, and I am struggling with it now as I write this book. I believe that my value to the universe is expressed mainly through my work. What I accomplish professionally is more important than what I have accomplished, or possibly could accomplish, in my personal life. I carry the question "Am I good enough?" Until recently, I felt no sense of contribution to the universe. I now know that what "I am" is more important than what I do. What I contribute to the personal growth of loved ones is more important than the lifesaving skills I learned in my medical career.

I am fortunate to have a vocation where I directly affect the welfare of others, but I now realize that helping others realize their God-given talents is more important than the application of lifesaving medical technology to my patients. There are many medical professionals who possess the same knowledge and skills I do, but there are only a few people with whom I am emotionally intimate and whom I am able to help by maximizing their innate talents. We all possess the ability to help others realize their potential through love, and the institution of marriage offers us the opportunity to do such work. All we need to do is seize this golden opportunity to give valuable gifts to our loved ones.

Dr. Lori Gordon in her book *Passage to Intimacy*[1] states that people with low self-esteem are unable to support the psychological and spiritual growth of their life partners. They are uncomfortable in intimate relationships, and have no sense about the origin of their dissatisfying intimate relationships. They often blame their partners for these feelings and for their sense of low self-worth, but the level of our self-esteem is set by our internal psyche. Our life partner may facilitate its enhancement, but the responsibility and the work of raising our self-esteem belong to each of us. Without this realization, we project the problems of our low self-worth onto our life partners and others. This can destroy relationships, and if it is repeated often, it can lead to a dissatisfying life. We need to raise our standards by changing our thoughts. We can make this improvement by changing our self-talk from "we should" statements to ones of "I will or I can." And if the word *don't* is part of your self-talk, delete it. This is important. Our subconscious mind cannot distinguish a positive statement from a negative one. Negative self-talk will lead you to doing what you state you don't want to do. We cannot avoid a "don't." It is one of the ways our minds work. The best illustration for this important point is the child sitting in a high chair with a cup of milk. His mother emphatically states, "Don't spill your milk." Now imagine what goes through the child's mind. He will automatically visualize the milk spilling, which greatly enhances the chances of its happening, just as his mind envisions it. We all tend to go toward what we think about. That is why self-talk works so well, and why the word *don't* doesn't belong in our vocabulary.

The correct parenting approach is for the parent to show the child how not to spill the milk by placing it in the correct place on the high chair and how to hold it with two hands to keep it level while bringing it up to his mouth. The positive approach will get the desired behavior from the child as well as your life partner. The only person you can change is yourself, but once you make the change, it will create changes in your loved ones.

Think Through Your Feelings

An important key to a successful loving relationship is learning to recognize your emotions. Linda certainly understands when she is upset, and she does not hesitate to talk about it. Most women do this better than men. I think the key to women's success in this important area of being conscious of their emotions is that they talk about them. Women friends often talk about their feelings, while men tend to talk more in action terms about sports, business, or politics.

When someone asks me, "How are you?" I usually respond that I feel fine. I automatically assume they are referring to my physical health, not my emotional state. Women, on the other hand, often receive a different message from the question. They may refer to their emotions as well as health. Women are more in tune with their feelings than men, and this may be exaggerated during pregnancy, when emotions can become intense.

It may be difficult for men to understand where all their life partner's emotional energy is coming from. We men usually react to our partner's mood swings by assuming that we are part of the problem, and that invariably leads to a defensive posture. This is not good for our self-esteem or for the relationship.

To correct this problem, I suggest two actions. The first is for my female readers to think through their emotions. Refrain from acting on them, without first trying to discover their origins. The second is to set time aside each day for your relationship with your life partner. This takes a commitment from both of you, and now is the best time to do it. Like so many of the exercises and suggestions in this book, the benefits from these learned skills will continue long after the successful completion of this pregnancy.

There are several useful techniques to help you think through your emotions. The first one is to write at the top of a page: I feel . . . Then relax and think about your feelings. Get into them; amplify and experience them to their fullest. Then let them flow on the page through your writing. If you are having a problem with writing, then I suggest that you try the technique for creative writing called "looping." This takes about twenty minutes. You will repeat the writing loop three times.

Set a timer for five minutes. Write at the top of the page, "I feel . . ." and then start writing as fast as you can, without making any corrections. Forget about spelling and punctuation; just write. Do not worry about what is going down on the paper. When the timer goes off at five minutes, read over what you have written and try to develop a grounding sentence that expresses what you gleaned from reading your first loop. Place the grounding sentence at the top of a fresh page and start the process over again. Then repeat it for a third time. Like sentence stemming, this is a powerful tool for self-exploration and will help you clarify vague feelings.

Writing tests the validity of your emotions, and amplifies your experience of them. Remember there is nothing wrong with experiencing emotions. Problems emerge when we inappropriately express or act on them. Your writing about them will help relieve the tension around these feelings, and help you think through them before acting.

If your emotions are about a loved one, write your feelings in a letter to them. Get them all down on paper. Read it out loud, and then write the response you would like to hear from your loved one. This can be very healing. It allows you to explore your feelings, safely express them, and then experience the healing response from the release of the pent-up negative emotion, whatever it may be. Remember, your unborn child shares all your emotions and the safe and effective expression of them helps you both.

You may or may not give the letter to the person who is the object of your feelings. The safety of making this decision after you write your expressive letter is a benefit of this technique. Once your feelings are on paper, you have time to cool down and reflect on the positive aspects of sharing what you wrote.

This technique of writing is important to men who tend to take action to solve problems. We are less likely than women to talk about our feelings. We will either retreat to think about them and cool off, or act without really considering the consequences. When men retreat to think and cool off, the women in our lives can do the relationship a favor by letting us go.

John Gray, Ph.D., the author of *Men Are from Mars, Women Are from Venus,*[2] describes men's retreat as "going into the cave." It is what we men do. It helps us control our emotions and behaviors. We will be able to talk better about our emotions after some cave time. So, in a heated argument, it is okay for men to ask for some cave time.

Like most men, when I become angry, I don't think well. After many heated arguments, I often remember the cogent points I forgot to make during the conflict. When this happens, I may feel the necessity to go back into the fray to make the point and by all means win the argument. When I feel this urge, I step back and relax, using deep breathing to try to get away from the male mind-set of winning the argument.

It is important for me not to worry about what I did or did not say. It is far better to concentrate on my feelings and what the other person is feeling. The quality of my listening skills is much more important in solving conflicts than what I have or have not said. I frequently have the urge to be correct, and this never solves a conflict. It is far more important to the relationship for me to understand my partner's point of view and reflect back her feelings using words that I understand. When I am able to do this, the results are likely to be positive. If I am left with anger or other important negative feelings after the argument, I use the creative writing technique of looping to explore and safely express my feelings.

Women, on the other hand, react to stress by talking. This is how they explore their feelings. They need to talk. Men must understand that their life partners do this to explore and understand their emotions. They are not necessarily asking us to take action. Men should resist the male urge to fix their problems during a heated discussion. We can serve our life partners and the relationship best by listening intently. Let your mind go blank and relate to the feelings expressed, so you can mirror them back to your loved one with your words and body. I recognize this is hard work for us men, but remember it is what love is all about.

An intimate relationship is not a license to freely emote negative feelings and emotionally abuse our spouse. It is a commitment to work on enhancing the quality of our partner's life. Partners in secure loving relationships are free from the fear of expressing whatever is on their minds, but with every freedom comes a responsibility. We need to respect our life partner as a unique individual whom we selected from all the people we know to help us learn life's valuable lessons.

What usually angers us about our loved ones is the very lesson we most need to learn. Use your life partner as a sounding board to help you become the person you always wanted to be, not a victim of your untethered emotions. I am not asking anyone to suppress feelings and thoughts—just the contrary. I am asking you to explore and express your most intimate thoughts and feelings in safe constructive ways. Always think about what is best for your relationship. Spiritual and personal growth require us constantly to evaluate our values, which entails letting go of ideals and convictions that may be dear to you. The institution of marriage is the best opportunity in life for our personal growth, and through marriage we nurture each other and our children.

It is not unusual for pregnant families to have stress in their relationship, and with stress we all regress to less mature behaviors that strain the marriage. Once we develop the emotional posture of helping our life partners be all they can be, we change our role of emotional victims to that of coach or trailblazer for our life partner. This small change in attitude pays great benefits to you and your life partner. At first there may not be much change in the behavior of you both, but with time you will notice changes in your relationship and in the contentment of your partner.

Each of us selected our life partners to psychologically fit our needs. Out of all the possible life partners we dated and courted, have you wondered how you ended with the one you did? It is no accident that you each selected one another. Remember the feelings of joy and invincibility you had when you first met your partner. Some think destiny selected their partner, and they married their soul mate. This may be true, but the psychological model that explains why we fight and get discouraged during marriage often helps us understand the reasons for the marital discord.

The life partner we select fills the suppressed parts of our personalities we lost during the early psychological development of childhood. That is why we feel so whole and complete when we are with them. They fill the lost parts of our personalities suppressed by our childhood reactions to the overdomineering parts of our parents' personalities.[3]

As an example, I am not as outgoing as Linda. She meets people and knows all about them; at the same gathering, I am more likely to withdraw and spend time in the corner of the room talking with a few select people. Her confident, and at times aggressive, verbal skills often irritate me, because I am more comfortable in familiar territory among friends whom I have known for a long time. My realization of what irritates me about her behavior is actually a part of her personality that attracted me during the courting phase of our relationship. I remember how happy I was when we went to a party where she easily fit in with a group of my friends. They instantly liked and accepted her. This memory helps me accept her aggressive verbal abilities when she is angry with me. Quite honestly I am verbally outgunned by her in any argument. I have never won a verbal argument with her, so I have changed my approach. When Linda is angry, I let her express her feelings and try to listen and convince her that I understand how she feels and the reasons she feels that way. This does not mean that I agree with her, but during the verbal exchange I don't try to convince her of who is wrong or right. I just go with the emotional content of the message and try to convince her that I understand why she is so angry.

More important for my personal development, I use her behavior as a guide for the parts of my personality that need maturing. My father had a forceful personality. He liked people and was outgoing. He behaved just like Linda does at a party. He worked the room and enjoyed talking with people. Unwittingly he suppressed this personality trait in me, and when I met Linda, I was drawn to the same trait in her. When we are together she represents the outgoing, affable part of our union. The personality trait I lost as a child is the one she possesses. That is why she makes me feel whole and wondrous when we are together. Our personalities mesh in psychological niches that benefit us both. Parts of my personality represent the suppressed parts of hers when we are together. You have the same relationship with your intimate partner. Think about it and you will recognize traits in your life partner that are similar to the dominant parent of your youth.

Try these sentence stems:

What I like best about my life partner is . . .

What angers me the most often about my life partner is . . .

Now review your stems and see if there are any similarities in the traits that both attract and repel you from your life partner.

What is important is to recognize that our lost personality traits are present in our life partner. The same trait that was attractive during courtship usually is the very trait that causes conflicts in our relationship. Linda's emotive verbal skills at times make me angry and lead to conflicts. When I am being attacked verbally and am at a loss for words, I get angry. During the confrontation, I work at remembering that this is the trait that I love and that first attracted me to her. What angers me is her use of the trait to attack me. My challenge during the heat of a verbal argument is for me to remember that the psychological fit that sometimes angers me also serves me in interesting and important ways.

The universal design for raising offspring throughout the animal kingdom of species of higher intelligence like mammals and birds is for it to be done in pairs. This is not by accident. Biology does not make arbitrary decisions. Parenting by pairs provides a biological advantage to the developing family. For us humans, this pairing gives our children the opportunity to absorb psychologically a larger variety of personality traits. Linda, my life partner, gives our children the opportunity to observe and learn from the excellent example her personality provides. They certainly will learn better verbal skills from her than from me. For me, Linda's interpersonal skills give me the lifelong opportunity to develop the suppressed traits of my personality that will ultimately make me a better person.

I use her behavior as a guide for my personal development. She also helps me with my spiritual development. The institution of marriage provides the most conducive environment to foster our spiritual and psychological growth. There is no better opportunity to grow and prosper spiritually and psychologically than in a loving relationship where there is the commitment to foster the unique qualities in each partner.

18

Selecting and Relating to Your Medical Team

If you refuse to accept anything but the very best,
you very often get it.

—*Anonymous*

Let's start with some sentence stems.

When I am faced with a problem . . .

I want a doctor/nurse-midwife who will . . .

I am happiest when . . .

I'm troubled that many patients don't do as thorough an investigation when they buy medical care as when they buy a car. If you're like most people looking for a new car, you systematically seek out the information you need to make the best decision about the vehicle you want and can afford. You shop around; look at various models; ask intelligent questions about its performance and the maintenance it requires; and possibly do some research on comparing the reliability and costs of owning the car before making a purchase.

The decision about which health care provider and facility you are going to use for your pregnancy is far more important than any car you will ever drive. My plea is for you to make a conscious choice to spend more time and put more thought into important medical decisions than most people put into planning a vacation or a major purchase like a car.

This chapter will lead you through a series of questions and checklists to make your "medical" shopping much easier while also taking into consideration some very important factors you might not otherwise have known even to ask about. But let's look first at the critical foundation that will influence all other choices you'll make.

Defining Your Role in Medical Decision Making

You may want to leave all of the decisions about your health care up to your health care provider. You may decide that he or she knows what is best for you and your baby. My patients frequently say, "Do whatever you think is best, Doctor." There is no question that my wife and I can make the best decisions about our pregnancy and what to do for our children, but as a health care professional caring for and about you and your family, I am not the best one to make those personal decisions. Medicine is not an exact science. There are many situations where there is not a simple correct answer. There are many different ways to do the same things, particularly in obstetrics.

Your value system is the best guide in making medical decisions. Why should your doctor or midwife make a decision about your health, your body, and your baby, when you have to live with the outcome of the decision for the rest of your life? Those of us in medicine have gone to school for many years and continue to study our specialty sciences in order to have the most current and accurate information, but that knowledge base does not give us the right to make your clinical decisions. We have a responsibility to give you solid information, but this is a task much different from making choices.

It's interesting to watch my colleagues make decisions about their own families' health, and then observe them interact with their patients who are trying to make health decisions. The processes are very different. We health care providers seek out the best information available, evaluate it, and then come to a decision about our family's health. When dealing with patients, most health care providers don't take the time to allow their patients to go through the same process that they go through in evaluating their own health problems. They use their clinical judgment to make quick decisions, which may or may not be the best decisions based on your value system.

Patients and health care providers should work as a team. Think of us as resources or consultants. Some clinical decisions are simple. For example, in a life-threatening situation when your fetus's heart rate suddenly drops during labor, it is an easy decision to deliver the infant by an emergency C-section. At the other extreme, in routine prenatal care it is an easy decision to perform important screening procedures.

But as the pregnancy continues, choices become more complex, and the guidelines are not as well established. This gray area is where you, your partner, your family, the people you respect, and your doctor or nurse-midwife need to work together. Remember, the goal is to select the best course of action.

For example, you may want to continue to work up to the time of the delivery, while your husband and family may want you to quit. Your health care provider may say it is okay for you to work, if you are willing to accept certain risks of going into preterm labor. There is no correct answer, and the best decision for each person will not be the same. You need to get good information about the risks involved, and then come to the best decision for you. Other examples where you will use your own decision-making capacities include exercise, sexual intercourse, diet, travel, and any medical problems that may arise.

Before you select a doctor or nurse-midwife, decide how much you want to participate in making decisions. Not clear about the degree of autonomy you want during your pregnancy? Here's a tip to help. How have you made major life decisions in the past, such as deciding how far to go in school, getting a job, getting married, having sex, and getting pregnant? If these life-changing events just happened to you, and you feel that you had little to do with the decisions that put you in your present situation, then you may want to select a health professional who will take charge of decision making, while you continue to play a passive role. On the other hand, if you were more active in making these kinds of life choices, you'll want a different relationship with your health care provider.

The same doctor or nurse-midwife will not be a good choice in both of these decision-making scenarios. Doctors and nurses have different communication styles and skills. Some of us want our patients to participate in medical decision making, others think they know best and want their patients to leave all the decisions up to them. Both types provide competent medical care, but your experience with them during the pregnancy and birth will be dramatically different. The chances of having a good experience are much better if you select a medical team that matches your style of decision making.

Asking a Friend

Many people ask a friend about which health care provider to use. However, most likely your preferences are not exactly like your friend's, and there is a good chance that her health care provider would not suit you. A recent study done by the American Medical Association shows that 70 percent of respondents agreed with the statement "People are beginning to lose faith in their doctors." In spite of this, most people rate their own health care provider highly. They must have either made a good choice in selecting their health care providers, or they are afraid to make a change because they don't know how to do it; or they feel loyal to their present provider of health care and don't want to disrupt the relationship.

Some good questions to ask your friends are:

Why do you like him or her so much?

What are the qualities that attracted you to their practice?

See if they made their decision based on the same ideals you would use.

Select a Birthing Facility First

Even before choosing specific people, however, first investigate the hospitals in your area. Find out which ones are the best in providing perinatal and newborn care and then select a provider who will admit you there for delivery.

A cautionary word about hospital referral services. Their recommendations on health professionals are based on the medical specialty requested and the geographic proximity of the practice's office to your home. They are primarily interested in building the practices of health care providers who use their hospital, which in turn helps their patient census. They usually employ a computer to generate a rotation system to recommend the next medical specialists in rotation. Clearly this doesn't take your value system into consideration.

Hospitals with good reputations tend to attract better providers of health care. They are highly selective in medical staff appointments, and they use their professional staffs to review colleagues in how well they do procedures such as deliveries and C-sections. A hospital wants to protect its reputation and does not want to expose itself to medical or legal liabilities. A hospital with an excellent reputation will have an excellent medical staff and is probably the best place to find good specialists, such as a neonatologist, if your newborn baby should need one.

Do some homework. If you have a friend who knows a nurse, or if you know a nurse working in the perinatal field, ask her about the hospitals in the area. Or call the medical editor of your local newspaper or TV station. Ask what resources are available in grading the quality of care given to obstetric patients in various area hospitals. Your state health department will have data on the number of deliveries, the percentage of C-sections, and the type of nurseries available in each birthing hospital.

I suggest that you choose a hospital with as many of these criteria as possible.

At least 2,000 deliveries per year

A neonatal intensive care unit

A C-section operating room in the delivery unit

A C-section rate below 25 percent

Twenty-four-hour coverage by anesthesia and neonatology services

I realize that the items I've listed are ideal but may not be available in your community, or may be limited by your insurance or transportation. Remember, *you* are still a more important determinant than the hospital you choose.

But the above criteria are far more important for the health and safety of you and your baby than amenities such as labor/delivery/postpartum rooms, steak dinners, and free limousine rides home that are advertised so readily in TV commercials.

I freely admit my bias against advertisements on television and radio. Any health care provider who has the minimal credentials and pays to be on the list of a medical referral system will be recommended by a locator service. Health care providers on a hospital staff, on the other hand, are more closely monitored by the hospital's peer review system than the cursory review done by physician locator services. Also, professionals on a hospital staff are monitored continually, and are expected to meet performance standards.

Ask Your Physician or Nurse Practitioner

After you have selected the hospital, the task of finding the obstetrical group, family practitioner, nurse-midwives, and pediatricians on the hospital staff that are best suited for you can be an even more difficult task. The easiest and best way is to ask another health professional. Typically they will give you several names and telephone numbers and send you off to do your own research, but this is a good start.

No health care provider will recommend a colleague he thinks is incompetent, but he may recommend one who has sent him patients in the past, or one with whom he wants to build a referral relationship. He will probably not spend much time thinking about which professional colleague will best meet your needs. If you want to participate in clinical decision making, a good question to ask is who delivered his or her children. If you don't want to be responsible for clinical decisions, ask for a medical team who will take charge of your health. In my practice, which is entirely by referral, I can tell which colleague sent me the patient by her style of relating to me. Patients tend to go to health care providers who have a communication style similar to their own.

Clinical Decision Making

Okay. So you've determined which hospital you want or is available to you. Let's now explore the steps to clarifying your values; information gathering, such as insurance coverage and convenience; and verifying your choice through interviews and personal experience.

Explore Your Values

We all have values that are the basis for our decisions and many of our actions. Often they're tucked away in the inactive parts of our conscious mind, but they're always at work guiding us in what we do and say. It is a good idea early in the decision-making process to shine light on these values, to declare them openly, and to rank them in order of importance.

Recognize that your values are part of your heritage, what you have grown up with or experienced during your life. You share them with your parents, friends, and other influential people in your life. You gravitate to people who have similar values. "Birds of a feather flock together" is a cliché but true. So, one quick way to describe your values is to look at the values of the people around you.

If you run with a racy crowd of friends who like fancy cars and expensive country clubs, then a material lifestyle is likely to be an important value for you. If you decide that you don't like these values, it is easy to change them. Make the conscious decision to do it, and it will happen. It may cause havoc with some close friends, but soon friends with values similar to your own will come into your life. Remember, your friends and their children will affect your child's future values.

Here is a self-exploratory exercise that will discover your values:

1. Write down as fast as you can all that you value in life. It might be important feelings, goals, possessions, and/or your relationships.
2. Put the list aside for a bit, relax, and clear your mind. (We'll look at a whole range of relaxation techniques in chapter 19.)
3. Review your list and make any additions or alterations to it. If something doesn't make sense, write it at the top of a fresh piece of paper, close your eyes, and visualize the word in your mind. Then begin to write again and you may find a more accurate word to describe this value.

Now it's time to invite significant others to do the same exercise.

Develop Your Pregnancy Support Group

Since your life partner, family, and close friends will have much influence on your developing fetus as well as your child, it's a lovely idea to ask them to go through the same exercise you just completed.

You are in charge of this pregnancy and each decision you make needs careful consideration. You will need the support of loved ones when you get discouraged, or if problems should arise. They also are important in helping you maintain discipline during the trying times of your pregnancy quest. They will celebrate with you on the peaks of your experience, and encourage you through the valleys. You are honoring them by including them on your quest.

At a group meeting, have each person rank his or her values in order of importance. Compile a list of everyone's top priority. Check those items that come up more than once. Continue this until all the values are listed.

Then, as a group, discuss the merits of each value and its ranking. This will help all involved clarify their own values, and it will be easy for you to see whose values you appreciate and who should be included in decision making. If you and your life partner have dramatically different values and are unable to reconcile differences, you'll have some work to do before the baby arrives.

Some people have found meetings like this to be heated and lengthy. You may want to choose carefully whom you invite if you know someone is inflexible or likely to try to sway everyone to his point of view, but most people are passionate about their values and that's okay. Let the energy of the discussion flow. Remember, this is a positive process that will help you make the best decisions for you and your baby.

Passionate people often express themselves with energy, which is sometimes interpreted as anger. Anger is okay in a loving relationship. Know that your love for the angry person is big enough to hold their anger. It is far better for all involved, including your unborn child, for the anger to be expressed openly and supported rather than suppressed.

Here are some examples of what you might discover from this process and what they mean to your decision-making process:

- If you have listed religion or your relationship with God as an important value, then you will need to find a doctor or a nurse-midwife who shares the same religious beliefs that you and your family have. You will need to include appropriate questions to ask during the interview process.
- If you value family and family relationships, then you need to find a health care professional who also values family life. He may be more tolerant of your family members' staying with you while you birth your baby.

- If you value money and saving it, you need to find an obstetrical practice that is efficient and interested in cost savings, and participates in your medical insurance.

*Interview Your Health Care Providers Before
Making an Appointment*

The next step is to ask your insurance carrier to send you a list of area health care providers and hospitals covered by your insurance. Call these establishments and start asking questions. Don't be embarrassed or hesitate to do this. Be assertive and confident, and at the same time be sure that you understand what they are saying. Ask questions until you are sure you understand their answers.

This positive assertiveness is different from skepticism, which can lead to conflict and lack of trust. You don't want to be a problem patient; on the other hand, you want to ask questions that engage your medical team and their office staff in a dialogue in which you both provide and receive information.

Here are some important things to evaluate:

- How quickly is the phone answered?
- How helpful is the person answering it?
- Ask the office manager about insurance coverage, the number of physicians and nurse-midwives in the group.
- What are their call schedules?
- What hospitals does the practice cover?
- How many partners does the practice have?
- Do they "cross cover" with another practice? (Two separate practices share covering the hospital and do deliveries for each other. In such a situation you may have someone attending your delivery whom you have never seen.)
- What is your health care provider's opinion of this book?

If the people on the phone or specific health professionals are uncomfortable answering these kinds of questions, you know that practice is not for you. If you have problems understanding what they are telling you, there may be communication problems in the future. If you feel timid about this interview process, bring along a member of your values clarification group, who can act as a spokesperson and help you evaluate the situation.

I also encourage you to visit the hospital, the delivery room, the postpartum unit, and the nursery. Call the hospital's administration office for an appointment with the clinical coordinator for obstetrics and the nursery. They should be willing to arrange a tour for you.

Here are some things to do and evaluate at the hospital:

- Talk with the nurses and other hospital personnel. Go into the family lounge on the obstetrical unit and ask questions of the family members there. Let them know you're not an investigative reporter, or someone with an official capacity evaluating the hospital's services—you are expectant parents just doing some homework on where you plan to deliver your baby.
- Do the health care professionals appear relaxed and not in a hurry?
- Do you understand their answers?
- Is the office or hospital area clean looking?
- Do the personnel act frustrated, or are they proud about what they are doing?
- Do you feel comfortable with them?

In this evaluation process, don't forget the pediatrician or family practitioner who will be caring for the baby. Call his or her office and go through the same process. The effort you put forth at this time will pay great dividends in peace of mind and efficient use of time in the future. Health care professionals should welcome the fact that you are interested in their background, experience, and competence. Remember, their national reputation is not as important to your health care as is how well you are able to communicate with them.

Get Background Information About Your Provider

Most health care providers are proud of their accomplishments and don't mind talking about them. Here are some things you want to know:

- Have they graduated from a medical or nursing school in the United States or Canada? These are all accredited schools. If they are a U.S. national by birth and graduated from a foreign school, you may wonder why they went offshore for their training, when there are so many good schools on our continent. A foreign national who graduated from a foreign school does not carry the same implications. Foreign schools vary in quality of training and foreign-trained medical students have to pass the same exams to practice medicine in the United States as American-trained physicians do, but their failure rate is greater.

- What is their residency training? A residency is extra training beyond the four years of medical school, and is not required in all states. Be sure that it is in the clinical field of obstetrics, pediatrics, or family medicine.
- Which hospital did they train in? It is a good sign if you recognize its name. You may want to call the hospital to be sure that the training program is accredited by the specialty board.
- Do they have further training in a subspecialty like maternal fetal medicine in obstetrics, or neonatology in pediatrics? This training takes another three years after completing the residency. Again, ask the name of the institution, for the same reasons as stated above.
- Are they board certified? Board certification means that the health care provider has passed an exam that demonstrates that he or she has a knowledge base recognized by a national organization as being important to the practice of that specialty. It does not necessarily mean that the medical professional is competent, or, more particularly, the best one for you.

Board eligibility is different from being board certified. A board-eligible physician indicates that the physician has only completed an approved residency but has either not yet taken the board exam or has failed it.

Finally, if you want to know about the number of lawsuits against the practice you are evaluating, or if you want to know if the state medical board has sanctioned the health care provider for any reason, you can call your state medical board for this information. My recommendation here is to leave evaluation of these important matters up to the medical staff of the hospital you have selected. They know more about these processes and how to evaluate them correctly, and there is very little bias or cover-up in most hospital credentialing processes.

If you are not satisfied with the medical team, nurses, or birthing hospitals that you have investigated, then widen your search. A consumer poll conducted by the Robert Wood Johnson Foundation ranked office location as the second most important criteria in the consumer's selection of a medical practice, just behind the health care provider's reputation. In spite of this popular criterion, I think it is better to travel extra distance to find the right birthing team than it is to put up with discomfort at a local facility.

I am assuming that you have decided which type of health care provider to use for your obstetrical care. I also assume that you are going to deliver in a hospital or a birthing center. I support the use of nurse-midwives. They are excellent with patients and seem to spend more time at the bedside with their laboring patients. If you choose to have a nurse-midwife team, I suggest that you evaluate the nurse-midwife team you select in the same manner as the physician team, but you will need to go a step further. All midwives practicing in a hospital are covered by a physicians' group during the pregnancy, and you need to evaluate them as well.

Another important question to ask is: Is there always a backup physician in the delivering hospital, or are they called from home? If called from outside of the hospital, what is the usual response time? I would ask about this important issue when you visit the delivery unit. The national standard is that an emergency C-section should be performed within thirty minutes of the decision to do it.

Home Deliveries

Being a neonatologist who cares for high-risk newborn infants, I have treated infants damaged by home births. In general I think it is best for a child to birth in a hospital or birthing center where unexpected emergencies can be handled expeditiously.

I recently had a nurse-midwife whom I deeply respect challenge my assertion that all births should occur in a medical facility. She gave me three excellent articles published in well-accepted medical journals that compare the safety of home births, birthing center births, and hospital births. These were large studies done by good researchers, and I was impressed with their study design, data, and conclusions. I presented these papers to a departmental journal club where all the pediatricians read and discussed the articles in detail. Like me, my colleagues in pediatrics were impressed with the quality of these research articles on this controversial issue. These articles and the journal club changed my opinion about the safety of home births, so I asked my midwife colleague if I could attend a home birth.

I have attended thousands of births during my thirty-three years of clinical experience. Not once did I feel the way I felt at my first home birth. During the home birth I felt I was intruding into the family fabric of an important, intimate life event. I was uncomfortable and wanted to leave so this intelligent, loving couple could have some privacy. They worked beautifully together as a team. They certainly were more comfortable, intimate, and open than the many couples I observed birthing in a hospital. They had more power over decisions and were able to exercise all their desired options, such as bathing or walking while laboring. Her husband was better able to comfort her with loving behaviors such as pillows, cuddle positions, back rubs, and requests for ice chips. The birth was a beautiful, personal family milestone.

If you choose a home birth, be sure that you are doing it for the right reasons. The guidelines in the clinical research articles for selecting a home birth were very strict. The births were all attended by a licensed nurse-midwife. Each patient was screened early in the pregnancy by an obstetrician who worked with the nurse-midwife and was familiar with the circumstances around birthing at home. If there were problems with the pregnancy or labor, the women were immediately transported to a birth facility. Such risk factors as preterm onset of labor, breech position, high blood pressure, poor growth in the unborn child, the presence of meconium (fetal fecal material) in the amniotic fluid, prolonged labor or membrane rupture, or fetal distress were all indications for a hospital birth.

19

Creating Fetal Love Breaks by Putting It All Together

The quality of a life is determined by its activities.

—*Aristotle*

It's time to train like a professional athlete. You are pregnant, maybe you have a career, a home and family to care for, and many other interests. You are in a time crunch. You are preparing to birth your baby. Your pregnancy is calling you to evaluate your values, control your mind, change behaviors, and accept new responsibilities. It all will culminate with the intense emotional and physical experience called labor. To meet these challenges you need to be at your best. Start now preparing for your ideal performance as world-class athletes do.

Let's look at two seemingly unrelated fields of science—psychology, as it pertains to achievement in the business world, and sports medicine. You may be thinking that you are not in the business world, have never trained for a sports event, and have no idea how to do this. It doesn't matter. There is much more to athletic training than physical exercise, and I, your trailblazer, will show you how elite athletes prepare spiritually, psychologically, and physically for their sporting events. The principles are the same if you are preparing for a business presentation, an athletic event, or for birthing your baby.

Some days you are smarter and stronger than usual. Events flow, you're on a roll. You may think these days just happen, but you will learn now how to prepare for maximal performance days. Most people who must achieve peak physical intensity and concentration know how to prepare for maximal performance. Certainly, you want to be at your personal best when you go into labor. Think of your pregnancy as a training period that will lead you to the goal of achieving a personal peak performance, a time when you will be mentally and physically fit to be your best to meet an important challenge. As with other skills you have learned in this book, peak performance is achieved by following an action plan.

Stephen Covey and others are leading an effective business revolution in America. The principles of management described in Covey's book *The Seven Habits of Highly Effective People* are thought by many to be responsible for the emergence of our nation's economy from the doldrums of the 1980s into the dominant world position it enjoyed during the 1990s. Two of his basic tenets are that an early investment in quality pays great rewards, and that one can improve his or her efficiency by doing what is important rather than what is urgent. By keeping your mind focused on what is important and having a clear idea of what you are striving to achieve, you become a more effective manager of your time and energy.[1]

Begin by having the end in mind. The more clearly you are able to define what you want to achieve, the more likely you are to be successful doing it. A pregnancy is composed of 280 days, punctuated by 40 seven-day intervals. You can begin today to build a successful pregnancy by completing a small meaningful step each day until, at the end of your gestation period, you accomplish your goal by stringing together the small steps you took one at a time. More about this in the section on goal setting in this chapter where I discuss the importance of a pregnancy mission statement.

Developing Passion for Commitment

Having a baby is a momentous life event. A good birth is the precious gift that lasts a lifetime. Yet pregnancy may be risky. By now you know the action steps needed to help improve its outcome. All you need is the passion to develop a plan and the discipline to follow it. In chapters 10, 11, and 12 you learned the importance of managing fear, developing self-esteem, and living responsibly. Now, your drive is to push through the tough parts of your pregnancy plan.

There is no greater motivator than love to help us work on difficult goals. Dear reader, you may be thinking that you know you will love your child but you don't love being pregnant. You may think it is unbecoming and inconvenient, and you don't know how to start managing all the behavior changes that can improve its outcome. Pregnancy brings families closer. There is a long tradition in societies of protecting and supporting pregnant women. Call upon your loved ones. Ask them to share their love with you—and expect it. You and your unborn baby deserve it. Remember the words of Robert Frost, "What is done well is done for the love of it, or it is not really done at all."

Begin by putting what is important before that which is urgent. Center your energy and thoughts into the present and focus on enjoying the process of changing your unwanted behaviors. Once you start, your trust in God and your ability to improve thoughts and behaviors will intensify. Remember the power of prayer and the important concept of the universe being friendly. Your responsibilities are to forgive yourself, forget the past, and to do your best right now. You will train to improve your spirituality and self-esteem. You will learn the importance of periodicity, the rhythm of intense effort interspersed with periods of relaxation. In fact, you may so enjoy being your best that you may use your newly learned skills and activities for the rest of your life. I know they will serve you well, and there is no better time to learn them than during pregnancy.

Striving for your best is risky. After all, you may not meet your expectations. Remember the work you did on facing fear and the words of Emerson, "Do the thing you fear, and the death of fear is certain." Just accept whatever now frightens you and don't fret about the outcome. Concentrate on the process you have set in motion and allow your changes to evolve. As you advance along the behavior change continuum discussed in chapter 14, you will start to love the process. Your love for your unborn child is easily transformed into loving the process of nurturing your pregnancy to the wholesome conclusion of birthing your healthy and happy baby. Once this happens, your passion to press forward will overcome any barriers that block you from achieving your goals.

Try making your pregnancy playful. Learn to laugh at funny little things that happen, like bumping into furniture or people, your food cravings, the change in your shape, or just feeling awkward. Remember, your baby shares your joy and sense of humor. Don't dwell on your limitations. Do what you can with what you have. Think about what brought you joy in the past and bring it into the pregnancy play frame. If you feel that you cannot laugh at your situation or that you just don't have the passion to do the work to change behaviors, look at the balance between work and rest in your life and at your stress level. Remember that these are manageable. Your goal is not to reduce stress or do less work, but rather learn how to rejuvenate yourself after work and manage your reaction to stress.

Managing Your Stress Reaction

Have your ever heard someone say, "I am under too much stress. I can't handle all this stress. If I could just get the stress out of my life, I would be happy"? Well, the only way to eliminate the stress in your life is to die. Life is stressful! You can change your job, inherit a million dollars, have perfect children, and your life will still be stressful. Once you accept stress as part of life, then you can stop trying to eliminate it and start learning to manage it. Stress has its good qualities. It helps us solve problems and achieve goals. Most people just live with stress. But during pregnancy, just living with it is not good enough. You must manage it.

In primitive times, when the stress response protected our ancestors from danger, they reacted with physical exercise. They either fought the danger or ran away from it. Our bodies still respond to stress by chemically preparing for physical activity. Now, in your world, fears both real and imagined (our bodies can't tell the difference) are always present, and our "fight or flight" response to stress stays prepared for physical action. We can't run away from nor can we physically fight danger like our ancestors did, so the stress neuropeptides remain in our bloodstream to do their damage. The only way to protect our bodies and your unborn child from this daily wear and tear is through disciplined practice of physical exercise and meditation—two good ways to ensure your health. (Remember what you read about the deleterious effect of stress neuropeptides on your unborn child in chapter 7.)

Modern life has not reduced stress. There is more stress in our lives as we face the compression of time and distance due to technological advances in communication and transportation. More and more events in the world are brought to our attention through communication media like television, faxes, and the Internet. We, in our daily lives, are expected to solve more problems in less time. As the world's problems are beamed into our living rooms each night, we are confronted with more and more violence, which builds fear. There is no respite from the continual stimuli that supercharge our metabolism into the flight or fight response, which, without exercise and meditation, leads to chronic stress and ill health.

You are probably thinking, "No one understands the amount of stress in my life, and if you had to deal with my circumstances and were not stressed out, then you just don't understand the mess I am in." The problem with this reasoning is that we assume that the external incidents in our lives cause our anxieties, when in reality it is not the events, but rather our attitudes and our responses to them. This is great news for stressed people! You can't control adverse events in your life, but you do control your reaction to them. You have the choice to be stressed or not to be. People have different reactions to the same experience. You may be stressed, while another person glides through unfazed. You may see differences in this respect between yourself and your life partner. The skills you are learning in this book will reduce the negative effects stress places on you and your unborn child.

Learn to Manage Stress

Any time you feel anxious, realize that it is imperative for you to recover from it. Elite athletes participating in sports events where there are short intervals of intense activity punctuated by periods of relaxation have learned the importance of periodicity—the concept of managing the periods of inactivity in ways that help them stay focused and properly prepared for their maximum performance during the next competitive activity. Pay attention to your body's stress level, and when it occurs make the commitment to recover from it by using self-care behaviors like exercise, yoga, and meditation. These three techniques help you recover from stress by changing your body's neuropeptide mix. Most highly effective people know from experience that self-care helps them achieve their goals and benefits the people they are trying to serve, so their rejuvenating routines become their priority. Learn from their example and make self-care a priority in your life.

To get the most from meditation, rely on your self-esteem and conviction that you are a unique part of the universe and able to overcome whatever predicaments arise during this pregnancy. I have had life experiences that at the time I thought were bad, but I eventually understood them as being good. These experiences give me the confidence to master crises that would have overwhelmed me in the past. I was better prepared to face the unexpected and tragic death of my eldest son, because I had learned from the sudden death of my dad to recall his wisdom and love in ways and at times that were not possible in our physical communication before his death. My self-esteem is based on my positive belief that the universe is safe and God loves me. I also have the commitment to magnify my faith through prayer, which I enrich with the following relaxation-meditation techniques.

What Is Meditation?

Meditation is the intentional concentration on a selected mental focus that reaches deep into our intuitive minds—the part that engages our physical and mental potentials for healing, joy, love, and peace. It is the oldest known method of stepping away from our controlling egos (which produce the negative self-talk that destroys our self-confidence) and toward a valuable resource: our inner wisdom. It puts us in touch with what some call our "supraconsciousness." Some may think they do not possess wisdom, but everyone does, and it is ready to help when called upon. The problem is that most of us have not experienced it, because we do not know how to activate the rich resources of our unconscious minds. Meditation will increase the power of your prayers, improve your mental and physical health and the health of your developing baby. It will change your life.

It may be difficult for you to believe that meditation can do all this for you, but I can remember learning in medical school physiology class that exercise conveyed no health benefits, and just ten years later our society went through the exercise craze. Now no one doubts the health benefits of routine exercise. I believe the next popular passion to sweep our society will be mental maturation, and I want you to be on the leading edge of this important self-help phenomenon. My goal is for you to develop good meditation skills and to use them for the rest of your life. Once you realize how helpful it is during this pregnancy, you will continue. Just try it. You will like it!

A recent prestigious medical journal showed that most of the illnesses and complaints family practitioners treat in their medical offices are stress related. It is well known that college students are more likely to get upper respiratory infections during exam weeks, and studies have shown them also to have low levels of interferon—an important mediator of our immune response to viral infections. You are less likely to become ill if you feel safe in your environment and don't drag your past fears into the present or, worse, project them into your future. Peace of mind is a key to wellness. To have true peace of mind you need faith, prayer, and good self-esteem.

In *The Relaxation Response* Dr. Herbert Benson convincingly proved, using modern medical research techniques, that meditation decreases our high blood pressure, heart rate, and oxygen consumption. Meditation changes our brain wave activity into restive alpha waves that are best described as a wakeful hypometabolic state, a physiologic antidote to the flight or fight response. Later studies by other investigators have shown that meditating for twenty minutes three times a week improves the natural killer cell and helper T cell activities in immune-deficient patients.[2] These research projects and many others clearly demonstrate that we have control over many of our body's functions that were once thought to be autonomic.

How to Meditate

There are many methods for meditation. The one described here was developed in the Western world and has the greatest acceptance in our society. This does not mean it is superior to other techniques, but it is the best one from which to begin developing your own method.

The simplest way to learn to meditate is to concentrate on breathing. Your body can live weeks without food and days without water, but only minutes without oxygen. Breathing is the most intimate and direct connection our brain has to the outer world. One fourth of the oxygen we breathe while resting goes directly to our brain. It is the one nutrient we consume that is not altered by a metabolic process before entering our brain cells. Other brain nutrients, such as glucose and amino acids, are packaged in foods that we alter by our digestion process before they enter our bloodstream to be transported to our brain. Other contacts with our world, such as light and sound, are changed into chemical form before they are transmitted along nerve paths to our brain. Oxygen is the purest contact our brain has with our environment, and this explains why breathing is so important to our mental state.

In feudal Japan, the samurai warriors practiced deep breathing for hours, as a major part of their preparation for war. They developed breath control to improve their archery skills during the stress of battle. Proper breathing techniques also helped them face their fears. Christian monks use breathing techniques during chanting to calm and center their minds for worship. Modern-day athletes use breath control to improve their concentration and athletic performance. These tools of breath control have withstood the test of time for centuries. Now you are learning their benefits.

Let's look at our language describing breathing, because it illustrates how breathing is tied to our emotions. You have heard these expressions: He waited with bated breath. I held my breath in anticipation. We enjoyed the breathtaking scenery. She breathed easily when finally out of danger. The artist was inspired [which can mean to inhale a breath] by the photograph to paint. The group conspired [which means to breathe together] to develop a plan.

A common term among athletes is "choking," which means the athlete was unable to handle the pressure of competition and his performance suffered. Sports psychologists who study athletic performance describe the "choking" performer's breathing as shallow and jerky. The athlete struggles to catch his breath. Athletes describe the feeling of "choking" as not being able to take in enough air. I remember having the same sensations when I had oral exams in medical school. I felt tense and nervous, but I was unaware of my breathing.

The next time you feel anxious, concentrate on your breathing and try the exercises described below. I wish I had this skill when I was in medical school; I know I would have made better grades. You will see Olympic downhill skiers taking deep breaths before their events or basketball players deep breathing before shooting foul shots. This helps them relax and work through "choking" to improve their performance.

You can control "choking" by learning to breathe like a newborn infant. If you have ever watched a baby breathe, you will recognize that he inhales by pushing his belly out. This facilitates the use of his diaphragm to inflate his lungs rather than the accessory muscles in his shoulders and between his ribs. Breathing with your diaphragm distributes the inspired air into the lower parts of your lungs, and gives you a much deeper breath, which aerates more lung volume. This increases the oxygen tension in your blood and ultimately enhances the supply of oxygen to your brain and muscles. In this way deep breathing relaxes muscle tension and improves mental and physical performance.

When you learn to breathe with your diaphragm, you will feel your energy surge with each deep breath. This is commonly called a cleansing breath. You then exhale by allowing the natural recoil of your lungs to gently release your breath through your mouth. During this gentle, passive exhale you will feel your muscle tension dissipate. By breathing properly you will break the "choking" response characterized by short jerky breathing.

Practice this deep breathing technique while sitting in a chair. Take a deep breath in through your nose while pushing out your belly. Slowly count from four to one while you inhale. At the end of inspiration hold your breath for a count, and then relax all your muscles while you breathe out passively through your open mouth. Once you have the slow breathing rhythm, try visualizing the numbers four to one in your mind's eye with each exhalation. See each number distinctly. Give each a soothing color. You can make the numbers bold and strong or graceful and fun. Play with this mental technique. If numbers don't work, then try letters. How about spelling your baby's name? Later you will start using mental pictures that have special significance for you.

It is easy to practice this breathing technique and a good way to relax quickly. Find a position in which you are relaxed but not asleep. You can either be in a chair with both feet on the floor and hands in your lap or in a supine position on the floor with your head slightly propped by a pillow. In either position, keep your back straight to facilitate breathing and your head in line with your spine. Then start breathing, using the described technique of diaphragmatic breathing. Place your hand on your abdomen, just below the rib cage, and practice pushing it away from your back as you breathe in. On exhalation, feel your muscles relax as you passively allow the air to escape from your lungs. After a while you will develop a comfortable rhythm. This simple breathing technique can be used at your office, at home, in your car while stopped in traffic, or in checkout lines in stores. You will soon feel your muscles release their tension and your energy increase as you practice this new skill.

Once you're comfortable with the breathing exercise, practice concentrating on the muscle groups in your body while taking slow, deep breaths. Start with your feet. Some people find it helpful to contract the muscles, hold the tension, and then relax them. You will know when you are doing this correctly, because you will feel the flow of warm blood into your feet and toes. Progress up your body, contracting and relaxing each muscle group separately. Start with your feet, followed by the calf muscles, the thigh muscles, and so on until you reach the top of your head. This should take three to five minutes, a long time when you are trying to concentrate.

Once this is complete, rest while concentrating on your breathing. Thoughts will come into your consciousness, but don't be concerned. Just picture them as white puff clouds drifting into and out of sight as they pass by. Do not be harsh or judgmental about your ability to have a blank mind. It will come with practice. If you have trouble with thoughts, then go back to counting or seeing letters in your mind. Remember that this is the best way to enhance your prayer effect, improve your communication with your unborn child, and manage pain during labor.

Adding Visual Images to Your Meditation: What You See Is What You Get

World-class athletes use mental imagery to improve their performance. They imagine themselves, under stress in game-winning situations, making the perfect shot. Jack Nicklaus, the great golfer, calls this "going to the movies." He visualizes his golf shot being perfect before he selects his club and addresses the ball. This technique will help you perform at you personal best during labor and delivery. You will mentally walk your way through your birthing experience and rehearse how well you are going to control your mind and body. By using your mind's eye and meditation techniques, you can "preplay" your birthing experience and make it as ideal as you wish.

Try this simple exercise. Close your eyes and, in your imagination, walk to the edge of the top of a fifty-story building. Imagine there is no barrier there, and you can place your toes beyond the building's edge. Now, look down between your feet to the pavement below. Take a quarter out of your pocket and drop it, watching it get smaller and smaller as it falls down the fifty stories. You may have the physiologic response of fear, but the reality is that you are sitting comfortably reading this book. Your mind and body reacted to just your mental image. Your mind does not know the difference between reality and imagination. That is why we enjoy movies so much, and why you can benefit from mental rehearsals.

The key to visualization is the use of all your senses in developing your mental picture. Practice may not make something perfect, but it does make it permanent. That is why mental imaging of the perfect outcome is so helpful. You can practice the perfect "preplay" every time, and that increases the chance of its happening during the event you are rehearsing.

Relaxation through meditation, coupled with mental imaging, is the most powerful way to meet your goals in any aspect of your life, be it birthing your baby, saving for your child's college education, or being successful at your career. Victor Frankl, the German prisoner of war, stated that he owed his life to his imagination. While suffering in Nazi concentration camps, he imagined how he would present his experiences to large audiences in the future. Many successful executives, who use mental imagery before presentations, say they owe their career prosperity to the skill of "preplaying" their success.

"Preplay" Your Pregnancy

Here are some important tips that will help program your brain during "preplay." Make your visualization an action scene in which there is movement. See the scene from your perspective. See it through your own eyes, not those of a spectator. This will help you feel the image and train your muscle groups to the proper responses. Studies of athletes practicing "preplay" have demonstrated that there is activity in the muscle groups used in the events the athletes are "preplaying" in their imagination.

"Preplay" the relaxation of your pelvis and the dilation of your cervix during labor. See yourself successfully finishing your task. Practice feeling confident birthing your baby. Feel your energy during the uterine contractions and yourself completely relaxed between them. Remember the breathing techniques that work through "choking" and are part of the meditation-relaxation response. Practice regaining your energy during the relaxation between contractions, and then focusing all your mental capacity on the task of getting the most from the uterine contraction, whether it be pain control or pushing.

You can also add positive talk to these exercises. Remember how to control your internal chatterbox. Make your statements "I" statements and keep them in the present tense, for example, "I am pushing my baby out. I am proud of delivering you vaginally. I love the feel of your hair and skin." Be creative with your self-talk. Make it wild and outrageous. Be forceful and exaggerate your statements. Try developing images with these words and work on how they make you feel during your "preplay." You will develop this skill. Do not give up on it. It will come with practice. It is powerful!

Train to Be in the "White Zone"

World-class athletes call the ideal performance state the "White Zone." They describe it as slow-motion action washed with surreal peace. In the White Zone, they have complete faith that they will prevail. Afterward they can't fully explain their exceptional performance, but they call it effortless. They state that their performance was controlled by something beyond themselves. The White Zone is a rare state of exceptional performance that athletes claim comes with relaxation, faith, and prayer.

The White Zone consists of three elements. The first is a state of relaxation. The second is high energy, and the third is complete confidence in performance ability. You can practice relaxation by meditating with the mental imagery of a place where you feel safe and relaxed. I use a beach scene, but you may use your childhood bedroom or being in the arms of your life partner. Whatever scene you use, it is important to fill your senses with your imagery.

When I think of my beach scene, I feel the warm sand giving my back gentle support under the sheet I am lying on. I feel the intense sunshine on my face and chest. I hear the surf and gulls, smell the salty sea air, and see the azure sky filled with small white puff clouds. I use every sense I have to help create a vivid image in my mind's eye. This intensifies the neuropeptide response of my brain and enhances my physical response to the imagery. I have rehearsed this scene so often that I can recall it at any time without going through the relaxation-meditation procedure and still get the same physical response. I use it when I feel myself get tense before an important meeting or when I confront a very difficult clinical situation that requires me to be at my best under stress.

You will also need a sanctuary—a place where you feel safe and refreshed. Your goal is to relax in the seconds between uterine contractions, so you can regain your energy and concentration for the next uterine contraction. You can use props to help build your "sanctuary." Some patients bring pictures or scented candles that remind them of their favorite places. Others have music they used during their fetal communication sessions.

Getting fired up with positive energy, the second part of the White Zone, requires a different technique. Think back to when you were excited while doing something pleasurable. This is different from being nervous or angry. I use the feeling I have when I go into the woods to photograph wildlife. I am so focused on the activity that I lose all sense of time or location. Once you pick the memory of being fired with positive energy, use the same techniques of meditation and imagery to build its intensity. With practice you will easily recall the emotions that put you into your White Zone of ideal performance.

The opposite of positive energy is the negative energy of fear, anger, or nervousness. Many people let go of their positive energy when things don't go well. A very small setback takes them away from their optimistic mind frame—what athletes call "tanking." Athletes who tank stop taking risks because of fear. They are unwilling to put themselves on the line for success because they are afraid of failing. The classic tanking statement is, "If I really wanted to do this I could, but I don't care enough to give my best effort." Tankers may also use laughter to get themselves off the pressure point of success versus failure. They try to demean the situation to reduce the risk of failure. This is another way of saying "I don't care enough to try," ironically making them feel safer.

You want to be in a high positive energy state when you go into labor and able to shift between high and low positive energy states in periodicity with your uterine contractions. High positive energy is pleasing and filled with enthusiasm, while low positive energy is calming and relaxing. These two energy states are in contrast to the high and low negative energy states characterized by the fight or flight metabolic state and the feeling of being overwhelmed. These two negative energy states are dangerous places to be when you are in labor or trying to do anything that requires your best performance.

Take time to reflect on your energy states when under stress for optimal performance. Do you tank? Try these sentence stems to help explore this important area of ideal performance:

I was in a high positive energy state when . . .

I can get into a high positive energy state by . . .

When I was in my high positive energy state I felt . . .

I was in a high negative energy state when . . .

I was in a low negative energy state when . . .

I was in a low positive energy state when . . .

I can get into a low positive energy state when . . .

I feel at my best when . . .

I take care of my energy when I . . .

When you become attuned to which of the four cells of energy you are in, you will begin to develop methods of getting yourself into the positive side of energy. Once there you will then learn how to use periodicity to refresh yourself, so you can continue being in the White Zone.

The third White Zone component of confidence can be triggered by remembering previous great performances. You may never have been in the White Zone—few have—but you can "preplay" confidence by bringing back mental images and feelings of your greatest hour. That might be a sports event, an academic achievement, a religious experience, or any other time in your life when you felt your proudest and most confident. Try to remember how you felt, how you walked, what you were thinking, and how much energy you had. Unfortunately, most of us already use this technique but to our detriment. We have powerful images of past "failures" and we re-create them over and over. Try now to make your successes more vivid and your failures and disappointments grayer and darker in your memory. It is a wonderful gift for you and your unborn child.

If you have a vivid image of failure, try this mental technique to help diminish its importance to your subconscious mind. First select a previous great performance and practice its mental image. Then bring back the image of failure, and in your mind's eye see it dim as it fades into the distance, while the White Zone image becomes brighter and larger. With practice you will feel your muscular tension and fatigue being replaced with relaxed energy and confidence.

When you go into labor you will want to be in your White Zone, but there will be surprises that might keep you from being your best. You may be frustrated by your labor experience. It is important to plan with your labor coach how you will recognize when you are tanking or getting angry. Work out a plan to use music, meditation, and mental imagery to bring you back into your White Zone.

You'll be receiving all types of information during this pregnancy, especially when labor starts. Some information will be bad and possibly unsettling. How you handle small setbacks will determine how successful you will be in maintaining your progress toward your goal. You can go into training now using relaxation meditation techniques to desensitize yourself against fear of failure or the pressure of delivering a healthy baby. You can "preplay" your worst fears and then imagine yourself handling the situation with great aptitude.

Useful Mental Images

There are several important images to use once you accomplish relaxation and mental imagery. Each achieves a different objective. There are several good books on mental imagery for pregnancy that can be purchased from your book dealer.

Building a Sanctuary

You will need the mental image of a place you feel safe. Think of positive memories and where you felt the most secure in your life, a place of comfort where nothing bad can happen. Remember to use all of your senses to fill your mind with the image, so it will have maximum impact on you and your baby. Practice being in your sanctuary, so when you arrive at the labor and delivery unit you can be mentally "transported" to your sanctuary for complete relaxation. The following prayer by Norman Vincent Peale helps me build a sanctuary: The light of God surrounds me, The love of God enfolds me, The power of God protects me, The presence of God watches over me, Wherever I am, God is![3]

Fetal Well-being

After relaxing, visualize the oxygen you breathe in as warm white light filling your lungs with healing energy that passes into your bloodstream and flows through your body. See the warmth radiating from within you, and then focus the light in your uterus and see it in your mind's eye circulating through your baby's body. This is a great exercise to do with music. After practicing this, pay attention to the change in your baby's movements. This could be the gift of the White Zone to your baby.

Cervical Dilation During Labor

You can visualize your cervix dilating with each uterine contraction. Ask your labor coach to show you how far your cervix is dilated and how large it must be before your baby can descend the birth canal. This gives you a mental picture of what your body is trying to accomplish.

A useful technique during the second stage of labor, when you have the urge to push, is to visualize your vagina from the baby's perspective opening up like a red flower under the warm sun. You can have your labor coach place warm compresses on your perineum to help with this image. Remember your breathing technique and mental sanctuary to break the "choke" and to relax between contractions, using the concept of periodicity. You will recover between contractions in your sanctuary, so when your next contraction returns, you will resume with your personal best effort—be it pain management or maximal pushing. You will be in the White Zone where you are relaxed and confident.

I have used both these techniques with women in labor who have been told by their obstetricians that they needed a C-section if their labor did not progress in the next hour. In most cases the mother, who was frightened by the prospect of the operation, was able to concentrate on her mental imagery and successfully dilate her cervix enough to push her baby through the second stage of labor to a vaginal delivery.

One of the best times to use meditation and mental imagery is after exercise. Most of us exercise because it is healthy and gives us a sense of well-being. Few see it as a way to relax and refresh our mind, but that is exactly what it does. It is important for you to exercise during your pregnancy, but talk it over with your health care provider before starting an exercise program. Be sure it is safe during your pregnancy. You may have a medical complication that precludes any exercise.

Exercise

The three important elements to a good exercise program are frequency, variety, and intensity. You need to exercise at least three times a week using a variety of activities built around a play frame to keep you interested and coming back for more. Finally, you need to monitor your heart rate to assure proper intensity of your workouts.

In early 1994, the American College of Obstetrics and Gynecology published a statement on exercise during pregnancy that greatly liberalized their recommendations about exercise intensity. It stated that pregnant women can maintain their level of fitness and there is no evidence for exercise adversely affecting the fetus.

I strongly suggest buying a heart rate monitor to monitor your exercise intensity. An earlier recommendation by the American College of Obstetrics and Gynecology was to keep your heart rate below 140 during exercise, but now they have loosened that recommendation somewhat. If you use the calculation for an aerobic heart rate target—220 minus your age in years, times 0.6—you will find that the 140 heart rate is in the aerobic range for your age group. If you want to calculate the safe upper limit of the aerobic heart rate for your age, change the formula's multiplier from 0.6 to 0.8.

The only way your fetus can dissipate heat is through the placenta, and this is limited by your body temperature; therefore you need to avoid exercising in extreme heat or using hot tubs and saunas. You may also find during the later part of pregnancy that your balance is affected by the change in your weight distribution, and you may have more joint pain due to the stretching of the ligaments around your joints. For these reasons it is best to do low-impact exercise after the fourth month of pregnancy in a cool environment. Swimming, stationary cycling, or moderate resistance training using weight lifting machines are appropriate for most pregnancies. My suggestion is for you to consult your health care provider and ask her for an exercise prescription that is suitable for your age, level of exercise fitness, and health of your pregnancy.

In spite of the limitations discussed, your exercise program during pregnancy is a gift to you. It will give you a sense of well-being, relieves stress, and helps with the mental exercises presented in this book. Bobby Fischer, the great world-champion chess player, went into intense physical training for his match against the Russians. After his victory, he was asked why he trained so vigorously for the match. His explanation is a classic statement for the mental benefits of being physically fit. He stated that the main reason he had beaten his Russian opponent was his physical fitness, which facilitated his concentration during the later hours of the match. Vince Lombardi, the legendary professional football coach, stated, "Fatigue makes cowards of us all."

You will be better prepared to fight the emotional and mental stresses of pregnancy and labor when you are physically fit. Your brain feeds on glucose and oxygen, and exercise helps your body maintain these important nutrients during times of intense stress or effort such as labor. Check with the hospitals in your community to see if they have an exercise program for pregnant women. Or you can check our Web site, www.prenatalparenting.com, to read about our exercise and yoga videotapes. We also have compact discs for guided mental imagery and selected classical music tapes for prenatal auditory stimulation. The Web site will also have periodic reviews on developments in the medical literature germane to this book.

Once you start, stick with it, because you will begin to feel the benefits in three to four weeks. Exercise releases endorphins, natural opiates that give you the euphoric feeling commonly called the "runner's high." This bliss helps you change unwanted behaviors. It is a mood elevator and an excellent substitute for unwanted behaviors.

While exercising, use mental imagery of little dolphins or newborn babies swimming joyfully through your body. Some pregnant mothers tell me about the mental image of their fetus playing and running with them. If you can carry these happy mental pictures into the exercise period, your mind and body will benefit more from the activity. We hold emotional tension in our muscle groups. You can disarm your negative thoughts and tension by working and stretching your muscles. Remember, the word *motion* is contained in the word *emotion*. It is good to meditate and do positive mental imaging during and after exercising, because these practices further reduce many physical and emotional tensions. People who routinely exercise state they can run away from their negative thoughts and return refreshed and with new perspectives. Albert Einstein stated, "Our legs are the wheels of creativity."

After exercising, your body needs time to recover. Exercise stresses our bodies and the repeated stress and recovery cycles teaches our bodies and minds how to recover from stress. A well-designed exercise program gradually increases the workload on your muscle groups, heart, and lungs. The gradual increase in intensity with adequate periods of recovery will improve your posture, likely reduce your chances of lower back pain, and, most important, give you the stamina and muscle control to deliver your infant efficiently.

You will need to give a new exercise program three weeks of regular workouts with increasing intensity before you begin to feel the emotional effects of the program. Interval training is a good first step in developing periodicity skills. Set your bursts of maximal effort to last about one minute and allow two to three minutes for recovery. This time sequence duplicates the periodicity of uterine contractions during intense labor. During the high-intensity period of interval training, concentrate on putting forth maximal effort. During the recovery period you will practice the mental work of staying focused and the deep breathing exercises to relax in preparation for the next burst of high intensity. You may not be able to physically train with the intensity of a world-class athlete, but you certainly can apply the mental aspects of sports training to prepare mentally, spiritually, and physically for childbirth.

Nutrition

Most physicians get very little training in nutrition during their medical school education. I am no exception. I had to learn about nutrition on the job. When I begin to talk to patients about nutrition I usually find their eyes glaze over, because they find it so boring, so I plan to make this section short and sweet.

Good nutrition during pregnancy is important. How you eat affects your baby's neurological development. Most parents know this, but some don't know how to go about improving their diets. My suggestion is simple. Start reading food labels. They are full of useful information. Don't let anything pass your lips without first reading the label. You will soon know the fat, protein, and carbohydrate composition of your diet. Your goal is to divide your calories into 20 percent protein, 30 percent fat, and 50 percent carbohydrates.

I know these recommendations, but I have never been able to figure out if I am eating the correct proportions, so I don't necessarily expect you to do it either. It is simpler to set the goal of increasing the amount of protein and complex carbohydrates in your diet without keeping close track of the proportions of nutrients in your diet. Just look at the food labels and buy only those items that meet or exceed the recommended proportions of nutrients you want to consume.

Stay away from the center aisles in the grocery. You will find better foods by becoming a perimeter shopper. The fruits, vegetables, meats, and dairy products are all along the walls of the store. When you venture into the center aisles you will be tempted by the packaged processed foods that usually contain more fats, sugars, and salt.

Simple sugars cause big swings in our metabolism. They give us a rush of energy that lasts only thirty to ninety minutes. Later you feel the "letdown" we often experience after eating a meal rich in simple sugars. The goal is to stabilize your blood sugar level by eating complex carbohydrates that do not cause the sharp rises and precipitous drops in blood sugar. When you look at the labels on food, you will find a section called Total Carbohydrates, which is broken down into Dietary Fiber, Sugars, and sometimes Sugar Alcohols. You will want to keep dietary fiber high and the sugars and sugar alcohols low. You do not need to avoid the alcohols. They are not ethanol, which is associated with fetal alcohol syndrome.

If you are going to eat a sugar snack, make sure that it is done during the time of day that will not affect your performance. It is okay to treat yourself to your favorite candy every once and a while, but please keep it moderate. You will soon learn how it adversely affects you. I have been able to drastically reduce the amount of simple sugars I ingest by paying attention to how they make me feel. After three weeks of abstaining from simple sugars, I no longer crave them.

Another guideline is not to consume anything that has more than 30 percent of its calories as fat. There are now many low-fat products on the market that make it much easier for us all to keep our fat intake down. During pregnancy you also want to increase the amount of protein you consume. Your protein source can be either meats or vegetables. Just set the goal to take at least 20 percent of your calories as protein.

An important way to improve your diet is to eat more frequently. Try eating your larger meals in the morning and at noon and reducing the amount of food you eat at night. Eating more calories during the time you are most active helps reset your metabolism so more of the nutrients consumed are metabolized and less are stored as body fat. Most nutritionists tell us that it is best to eat six meals a day. Try high-protein snacks during your midmorning and midafternoon breaks. This will reduce the wild fluctuation in blood sugar levels that cause mood swings and loss in efficiency.

If you work, serve fruit juice and nuts instead of coffee and sweets as a snack for the next midmorning and/or midafternoon meeting. Then observe the difference in the group's interaction and productivity. You will be amazed at the change in behaviors. Your co-workers' behaviors will become your own laboratory to observe the powerful effects foods have on us.

It is a good idea for you to start thinking of foods as drugs and to try to determine the connection between them and your mood and energy level. You will be amazed at how much you can learn about nutrition by following these simple suggestions. Doing this work will become easier with time and practice. Remember that it is important work and a wonderful way to express your love for your unborn child.

Developing Your Pregnancy Mission Statement

A major component of putting it all together is goal setting. In chapter 12, you read that goals keep you focused on breaking through the inevitable roadblocks presented by your busy life. Setting demanding goals and following your progress toward them are strong motivators for changing behaviors—the key to prenatal parenting. If you have not already done so, now is the time to set goals that stretch your self-image. Make these goals so demanding that once obtained, your self-esteem will soar. Write down your goals and the reasons why they are important to you. Remember Thomas Edison's statement while trying to invent the light-bulb, "I would much rather fail in the pursuit of a demanding worth-while goal than to just by chance succeed at a lesser one."

The link between goal setting and success is well recognized. It started with the Egyptians and has continued down through the ages as an excellent management tool. Big corporations spend thousands of dollars on consultants who help them develop mission statements, goals, and objectives with action steps along a time line. They invest this kind of money because it works. The process focuses your energy and attention on what is important rather than on what is urgent and aids in making the difficult choices you frequently face during your busy day.

Fear is a common motivator, but not a healthy one. It adversely affects your health and that of your fetus. Commitment and love are the positive motivators that better serve you, but few people set goals based on them. You need to look deep into yourself to discover what is truly important to you. Now is a good time to review the sentence stems on self-esteem you wrote in chapter 11 to focus your attention on the com-pelling ideals you discovered for this pregnancy. The key is your vision of a successful pregnancy and how you translate it into goals and action steps. Do you truly feel competent to achieve the goals you have set? If not, then please reassess the areas in my book that you left unfinished.

A key to goal setting is not to postpone your happiness to the day you achieve your ideal. You need to find joy and the sense of accom-plishment in moving toward your planned objectives. You will have more pleasure in working toward your goals if you orient them to the new behaviors you want rather than to the pregnancy outcome. You have more control over behaviors than you do over outcomes; there-fore, you are better able to achieve them.

For example, attitude is certainly under your control. A good tar-get is to have the positive expectation of the power of self-talk, prayer, and faith. If you have the faith that prayer is powerful, it most likely will be. If your objective is to take a fetal love break three times a day, you are more likely to be successful than if you set a goal to have a vaginal birth with no pain medication. You may have the ambition of a "natural childbirth," but this plan is out of your control. There are too many variables over which you have no control, such as the nursing and medical policies of your birthing place, be it a hospital or birthing center. However, you can improve your chances for "natural child-birth" by being mentally and physically prepared to give your best effort toward achieving it.

You are probably in a childbirth class, and you may have written a birthing plan that lists your preferences during the birth process. You may intend to present your plan to your health care provider, who may or may not take it seriously. It is okay to have birthing preferences, but it is far better to have a pregnancy mission statement. This will be the standard by which you can judge all your activities and those of your life partner and health care providers during this pregnancy. It will be your beacon to guide you and all those who are trying to help you have the pregnancy outcome you wish.

It must be based on principles that empower you to make difficult decisions based on your ideal. If you have the feeling of meaningless-ness or emptiness in your life, then developing a personal life mission statement will quickly correct this and will set you on a course toward fulfilling your dreams. To do this effectively you will return to the sen-tence stems and other self-exploratory work you did to discover your security, wisdom, and power. This is the essence that defines you. A pregnancy mission statement should contain all that is uniquely you, what you want during your pregnancy, the birthing experience, and the rest of your life with your newborn child.

In writing the mission statement, list what is important to you and what you want people to remember of you. My dad asked me when I graduated from college to write my epitaph. I thought it was a strange request. I had no thoughts of dying. After all, I had too much to live for. My first draft was long and very ambiguous, but as the years passed, and I became more focused in my life, my values became clearer. Now my epitaph is my personal life mission statement. It describes me so well that I have stated in my will that it be on my tombstone. I want to be remembered by the words, "A man who loved God and the life He gave him." With this simple statement, I have my life beacon to guide me through all my decisions. When I feel my values are fraying, I refer to my mission statement that grounds my thinking so that I make deci-sions based on principles correct for me.

Your pregnancy mission statement can be your beacon for decision making. Reflect back to the exercise on values clarification in chapter 18 and write those values into your mission in concise statements. As your pregnancy progresses, your life will become more complex, and you will begin to feel time compression. When this happens, your pregnancy mission statement will bring you back to what is important. Stephen Covey suggests that individuals not only have a personal mission statement, but that families develop one too. Setting goals, describing action steps, and developing time lines becomes much easier with practice.

When you finish this process your life will change. You will no longer be reacting to life's predicaments. You will be making decisions based on your mission statement. Your friends will notice that your life has direction and an important purpose that brings you excitement and commitment.

Successful people who use goal setting state that writing down their dreams and setting up action steps along a time line is an enjoyable process. It's a great morale booster. When they progress along their time line of action steps, their self-esteem soars, filling them with positive energy. Of course, we are not always successful. At times we fail to meet the deadline of an action step, but this does not divert us from moving toward our ideal. The progress we made before being thwarted can be used to enhance our self-esteem and drive to persevere through the frustrating obstacles. When you meet adversities, renew your enthusiasm and dedication by reviewing your mission statement of love and commitment for your unborn child and family. Remember, it is much easier to renew your commitment when you are striving for a behavior change or a personal quality rather than an expected outcome of your pregnancy.

Getting Started

Big question: Where do you find the motivation to start? For example, your mission statement may contain the ideal of eating and exercising correctly. You set goals to exercise daily, following the guidelines of your health care provider, and to eat five healthy meals a day for the rest of this pregnancy. You then can use your appointments with your health care provider as milestones on a time line to measure your progress toward these goals. You could begin by writing down on paper, "During the next 14 days I will exercise seven times for 20 minutes with a target heart rate of 120 beats per minute." The next step may be to schedule the exercise times with yourself until your next pregnancy checkup, and the final step could be to keep track of your ability to follow through with your goals.

I commonly hear my patients complain, "My life is so busy that I don't have time to do the things I know are important. I am too busy doing what has to be done now." Many people feel that their lives are out of control. These patients are responding to what is urgent rather than to what is important. Specific goals attached to a mission statement set your priorities and help you answer the question: Is this the best use of my time? If you feel a time crunch, then start by taking small steps that give you immediate rewards for doing something worthwhile for you and your unborn child. (Please see the section on time management later in this chapter for more information on finding time for your pregnancy.)

Remember that success is not a competition. Don't measure your success by the feedback or approval of others. There are many people who outwardly appear successful but personally are failures, because they have not reached their potential. Success is not being the best among your peers. Success is doing your personal best. The important part of goal setting is the contract you make with yourself. Don't demean yourself if you fail this exercise. Remember, in failure there is always a learning process that will help you with your next attempt. As long as you keep trying you will never be a failure. It is far better to try and fail at a goal than not to try at all.

Why Do So Few Set Goals?

If goals can do what they did for the 1953 graduates of Princeton University, as discussed in chapter 12, then why don't more people use goal setting to improve their lives? There is no doubt that goals work. A few of the common reasons for not setting goals are discussed below. Read on and see if any of them explains why you have not used goal setting in your personal life.

You may think that you have done well during your life without setting goals. This is a very convenient and popular idea. When you don't have a mission statement, you are stating that life is easy and whatever happens is okay. You are leaving the future to chance, and you will live with the consequences. I disagree with this complacent attitude. Not having a life mission is like a sailing ship leaving the harbor and allowing the wind direction to dictate her destination. This may be the easy way to leave the harbor, but it is not an effective way to sail a ship. She is likely to remain adrift in the middle of the ocean for the rest of her existence. Without goals, you are setting your life adrift with little chance of achieving happiness and prosperity. With goals you set your life on course to bring about what you believe is important.

I commonly hear people say they have goals, but they keep them in their heads and do not write them down. Without a written goal, your thoughts are just wishes that you will try to achieve sometime in the future when you have time. This leads to procrastination and diminished self-esteem, a common and unfortunate way to live life, and a complete waste of your God-given talents. This attitude robs you of so much joy and excitement. The plan and action steps you set along a time line will increase your enthusiasm and excitement to such high levels that you will repeat the process over and over. You will ask yourself, Why haven't I done this before?

Birthing is a major quest, one that is worthy of bringing forth all of your talents and skills. Developing a mission statement and setting goals is the way to discover and use your talents. It will improve your health and that of your unborn child. Remember to write your goals down and break them up into measurable steps. Arrange the action steps on your daily planner or around your medical appointments so you will have a sense of urgency to accomplish them. Your mission statement needs to be consistent with your belief system. Setting high ideals and achieving them is the highest adventure on earth.

Managing Time

When are you going to do all the work suggested in this book? Setting goals may take time you think you don't have in your busy schedule. You can't reach all of your goals at once. You have to manage them through the medium of time. So where are you going to find the time?

You start by being a time watchdog. Try to budget it like you do money. It's interesting that most of us learn how to manage money, but few know how to manage time. We can get promoted to earn more money. We can borrow it, save it, or invest it. What is interesting about time is that we all have the same amount of it. It is universally distributed. There is no way to bank it, invest in it, or borrow it. When it passes, it can't be retrieved. That makes it more precious than money. I think of time as my most important resource next to my health, but I know much more about staying healthy and handling money than I do about managing time.

How do some people get more done during the day when all of us have the same amount of time? Those who accomplish more have learned the important life skill of being effective, which is different from being efficient. Some can get a job done in less time by doing it less well, but they are usually not as effective. In the long run inept people spend more time correcting what was done incorrectly in the first place. It is far more important to be effective and to go for quality than to be efficient. If you don't have the time to do it right the first time, then when do you think you will find the time to do it over? The way to be more effective is to schedule time to reflect on your goals and progress along your set time line. You will be better guided by using specific, demanding goals that are easily measurable along your time line. Please set a goal to manage your energy levels. This will keep your energy in the positive side of the balance sheet and will keep you away from chronic stress and fatigue that are so destructive to both you and your unborn child.

I believe effective people learn to make decisions early in the process. They are willing to take a risk to get started and modify the plan as they go. It is far better to take risks early in achieving a goal. This is true in investing for a retirement nest egg as well as setting time management goals. All champions were beginners when they started and most of them risked playing the fool early in the game to achieve their goal of championship status. Champions continually strive to be at their best by using the skills discussed in this book. They have the expectation of achieving their goals and are willing to pay the price.

A way to get control of your time is to be conscious of the time you waste. Write a daily log. This is like checking your expenses against a budget. Most people who take the time to write a time log find out that there are many hours during the day that can be used more efficiently. You can stop wasting time. Remember to do what is important rather than what is urgent.

There are times when the important thing to do is to recover from the stress of doing what is urgent even when faced with doing other urgent tasks. It is also important to reassess your goals each quarter to be sure that they are still in the proper rank of importance as stated in your mission statement. Plan your pregnancy backward, from the birth of your child at term to where you are right now. Take the risk early in the pregnancy to set goals to change behaviors. Develop a plan and take bold steps toward achieving it. Start now. Do not waste any more time. It is too precious.

Take a Fetal Love Break

Now is the time to accept the responsibility of giving your unborn child the gift of unconditional love that only you can give. Contract with yourself to start with a positive mind-set, write an exciting mission statement, set some challenging goals, develop action steps and a time line. Then commit to start now to learn to rely on your beliefs, develop the habits of prayer and positive self-talk, conquer your fears, enhance your self-esteem, and finally practice meditation and mental imagery.

Make the decision to take a fifteen-minute fetal love break three times a day. Structure the time around your personal and professional schedules. The first few fetal love breaks may be for writing down your goals or finishing the assignments in the previous chapters. Later you can use them to exercise, to eat a healthy snack, or to practice a new mental skill such as prayer. Just get started and make the fetal love break a habit. It will serve both you and your unborn child well.

As you work through the steps in this book, you will create new uses for your fetal love breaks. Early in the pregnancy you may be working on changing risky behaviors such as your negative internal chatterbox, not eating correctly, or not exercising regularly. Later you will practice relaxation and mental imagery to communicate with your unborn child and prepare for being mentally and physically ready for labor.

Psychologists have taught us that it takes twenty-eight days to develop a new habit. The challenge is to rid ourselves of old unwanted behaviors and replace them with new beneficial ones. You have read about successful techniques to help you do this and how world-class athletes use regimented behaviors and thought patterns to attain high energy states. The more ritualistic you are the more likely you are to be successful. Professional tennis players have rituals they use before matches and between points during the match. It does not matter what has happened during the last high-intensity period of play. They always prepare for the next point in the same way. This keeps them from falling apart in tight matches. They handle the recovery period between points with self-talk and diaphragmatic breathing. They use "preplay" and mental sanctuaries to help them get into the high positive energy state for the next point. After the play is over they quickly shift into low positive energy state by using rituals of diaphragmatic breathing and mental imagery. All this helps them prepare for their best performance.

Life, like a tennis match, is the pulsation between stress and recovery. If you feel stressed, your life is out of balance and you are not taking enough time for recovery. Change your attitude to look at problems as challenges that open new opportunities. With proper attitude and balance between stress and recovery, your motivation, energy level, and spirit will soar. Your confidence will be sky-high and your powers of concentration will be stronger than ever. When you begin to experience this, celebrate your victory. You are on your way to taking charge of your pregnancy outcome.

Remember, there are no failures during this pregnancy, just learning opportunities. Take each action step one at a time, with your mind set on your goal. Build new habits to carry you to your goals. Both you and your unborn child are projects in progress. In times when I am challenged by life events, I am reassured by Christ's words, "So I tell you, whatever you ask for in prayer, believe that you received it, and it will be yours."[4]

Notes

Preface

1. Children's Defense Fund, *The State of America's Children* (Washington, D.C.: Children's Defense Fund, 1997).
2. *The Future of Our Children,* The David and Lucile Packard Foundation.

1 Take a Fetal Love Break

1. Rima Shore, *Rethinking the Brain: New Insights into Early Development* (New York: Families and Work Institute, 1997); David Chamberlain, Ph.D., *The Mind of Your Newborn Baby* (Berkeley, Calif.: North Atlantic Books, 1998); Robin Karr-Morse and Meredith S. Wiley, *Ghosts from the Nursery: Tracing the Roots of Violence* (New York: Atlantic Monthly Press, 1997); Thomas Verny, M.D., and John Kelly, *The Secret Life of the Unborn Child* (New York: Dell, 1994).
2. Alison Gopnik, Ph.D., Andrew Meltzoff, Ph.D., and Patricia Kuhl, Ph.D., *The Scientist in the Crib: Minds, Brains, and How Children Learn* (New York: William Morrow, 1999).
3. Karr-Morse and Wiley, *Ghosts from the Nursery.*
4. Nathaniel Branden, M.D., *"If You Could Hear What I Cannot Say": Learning to Communicate with the One You Love* (New York: Bantam Books, 1985).

2 Communicating with Your Unborn Child

1. Robin Karr-Morse and Meredith S. Wiley, *Ghosts from the Nursery: Tracing the Roots of Violence* (New York: Atlantic Monthly Press, 1997).

2. John 1:14, New International Version (Wheaton, II.: Tyndale House Publishers, Inc.).

3. H. Als, G. Lawhon, F. H. Duffy, et al. (1994), "Individualized Behavioral and Developmental Care for the Very Low Birthweight Preterm Infant: Medical and Neurofunctional Effects." *JAMA* 272: 853–58.

4. Alison Gopnik, Ph.D., Andrew Meltzoff, Ph.D., and Patricia Kuhl, Ph.D., *The Scientist in the Crib: Minds, Brains, and How Children Learn* (New York: William Morrow, 1999).

5. H. Als, F. H. Duffy, and G. B. McAnulty, "Longterm Effects of Very Early Individualized Developmental Care in the NICU to 3 and 7 Years Post Term" (in preparation).

6. Robin Karr-Morse and Meredith S. Wiley, *Ghosts from the Nursery: Tracing the Roots of Violence* (New York: Atlantic Monthly Press, 1997).

7. Candace B. Pert, Ph.D., *Molecules of Emotion: The Science Behind Mind-Body Medicine* (New York: Simon & Schuster, 1997).

8. Gopnik, Meltzoff, and Kuhl, *The Scientist in the Crib.*

9. R. Kotulak, *Inside the Brain: Revolutionary Discoveries of How the Mind Works* (Kansas City, Mo.: Andrews McMeel Publishing, 1997).

10. Pert, *Molecules of Emotion.*

11. Peter W. Nathanielsz, M.D., Ph.D., *Life in the Womb: The Origin of Health and Disease* (Ithaca, N.Y.: Promethean Press, 1999).

12. Ibid.

3 On Becoming a Brain Architect

1. R. Kotulak, *Inside the Brain: Revolutionary Discoveries of How the Mind Works* (Kansas City, Mo.: Andrews McMeel Publishing, 1997).

2. Ibid.

3. Rima Shore, *Rethinking the Brain: New Insights into Early Development* (New York: Families and Work Institute, 1997).

4. Robin Karr-Morse and Meredith S. Wiley, *Ghosts from the Nursery: Tracing the Roots of Violence* (New York: Atlantic Monthly Press, 1997).

5. R. Kotulak, *Inside the Brain.*

6. Richard M. Restak, M.D., *The Infant Mind* (Garden City, N.Y.: Doubleday & Company, Inc., 1986), 56.

4 Fetal Development of Senses

1. David Chamberlain, Ph.D., *The Mind of Your Newborn Baby* (Berkeley, Calif.: North Atlantic Books, 1998).

2. R. L. Fantz (1963), "Pattern Vision in Newborn Infants." *Science* 140: 296–97.

3. T. G. R. Bower, *The Rational Infant: Learning in Infancy* (San Francisco: W. H. Freeman, 1989).

4. Don Campbell, *The Mozart Effect: Tapping the Power of Music to Heal the Body, Strengthen the Mind, and Unlock the Creative Spirit* (New York: Avon Books, 1997).

5. Chamberlain, *The Mind of Your Newborn Baby.*

5 The Intrauterine Temple of Learning

1. David Chamberlain, Ph.D., *The Mind of Your Newborn Baby* (Berkeley, Calif.: North Atlantic Books, 1998).

2. Daniel Goleman, *Emotional Intelligence: Why It Can Matter More Than IQ* (New York: Bantam Books, 1997).

3. Robin Karr-Morse and Meredith S. Wiley, *Ghosts from the Nursery: Tracing the Roots of Violence* (New York: Atlantic Monthly Press, 1997).

4. D. H. Hubel (1982), "Evolution of Ideas on the Primary Visual Cortex, 1955–1978: A Biassed Historical Account" (Nobel lecture). *Biosci Rep* 2(7): 435–69.

5. F. A. Campbell and C. T. Ramey (1994), "Effects of Early Intervention on Intellectual and Academic Achievement: A Follow-up Study of Children from Low-Income Families." *Child Development* 65: 684–98.

6. A. DeCasper and M. J. Spence (1986), "Prenatal Maternal Speech Influences Newborns' Perception of Speech Sounds." *Infant Behavior and Development.* 9: 133–50.

7. Alison Gopnik, Ph.D., Andrew Meltzoff, Ph.D., and Patricia Kuhl, Ph.D., *The Scientist in the Crib: Minds, Brains, and How Children Learn* (New York: William Morrow, 1999).

6 Intrauterine Emotional Development

1. H. A. Weisman and G. A. Kerr, *Fetal Growth and Development* (New York: McGraw-Hill, 1970).

2. Robin Karr-Morse and Meredith S. Wiley, *Ghosts from the Nursery: Tracing the Roots of Violence* (New York: Atlantic Monthly Press, 1997).

3. G. W. Kraemer, "Social Attachment, Brain Function, Aggression and Violence," *Unlocking Crime: The Biosocial Key,* A. Raine, D. Farrington, P. Brennan, and S. Mednick, eds. (New York: Plenum Publishing).

4. C. Darwin, *The Expression of the Emotions in Man and Animals* (New York: The Philosophical Library, 1955).

5. Candace B. Pert, Ph.D., *Molecules of Emotion: The Science Behind Mind-Body Medicine* (New York: Simon & Schuster, 1997).

6. S. McCarthy and J. Moussaieff, *When Elephants Weep: The Emotional Lives of Animals* (New York: Delta, 1996).

7. Robin Karr-Morse and Meredith S. Wiley, *Ghosts from the Nursery: Tracing the Roots of Violence* (New York: Atlantic Monthly Press, 1997).

7 Emotional Communication with the Unborn Child

1. Candace B. Pert, Ph.D., *Molecules of Emotion: The Science Behind Mind-Body Medicine* (New York: Simon & Schuster, 1997).

2. Robin Karr-Morse and Meredith S. Wiley, *Ghosts from the Nursery: Tracing the Roots of Violence* (New York: Atlantic Monthly Press, 1997).

3. Clark and Schneider (1993), "Prenatal Stress Alters Social and Adaptive Behaviors in Adolescent Rhesus Monkeys." *Developmental Psychobiology* 26(5): 293–304.

4. H. Als, F. H. Duffy, and G. B. McAnulty, "Longterm Effects of Very Early Individualized Developmental Care in the NICU to 3 and 7 Years Post Term" (in preparation).

5. T. B. Brazelton, *Touchpoints: Your Child's Emotional and Behavioral Development* (Reading, MA: Addison-Wesley Publishing, 1992).

6. David Chamberlain, Ph.D., "Transpersonal Adventures in Prenatal/Perinatal Hypnotherapy, *Transpersonal Hypnosis,* E. Leskowitz, ed. (Irvington Press, 1997).

7. A. N. Schore (1996), "The Experience-Dependent Maturation of a Regulatory System in the Orbital Prefrontal Cortex and the Origin of Developmental Psychopathology," *Development and Psychopathology* 8: 59–87.

8. A. Raine, *The Psychopathology of Crime: Criminal Behavior as a Clinical Disorder* (New York: Academic Press, 1993).

8 Choosing the Road to Birthing a Healthy Baby

1. P. Glynn, *God, the Evidence: The Reconciliation of Faith and Reason in a Postsecular World* (Roseville, Calif.: Prima Publishing, 1999).

2. Ibid.

3. F. Hoyle, *The Origin of the Universe and the Origin of Religion* (Wakefield, R.I.: Moyer Bell, 1993).

4. V. Nabokov, *Pale Fire,* as quoted by Larry Woiwode in "Not Fading to Nothing," in *Books & Culture,* November/December 1995.

5. P. Morrison and the Office of Charles and Ray Eames, *Powers of Ten: About the Relative Size of Things in the Universe* (New York: W. H. Freeman, 1994).

6. V. Frankl, *Man's Search for Meaning* (New York: Pocket Books, 1963).

7. A. H. Maslow, *Motivation and Personality* (New York: Harper and Row, 1954).

8. J. Campbell with B. Moyers, *The Power of Myth* (New York: Doubleday, 1988).

9. K. Gibran, *The Prophet* (New York: Alfred A. Knopf, 1923).

9 Faith, Prayer, and Love

1. L. Dossey, M.D., *Healing Words: The Power of Prayer and the Practice of Medicine* (San Francisco: HarperSanFrancisco, 1993).

2. Ibid.

3. R. Rosenthal, "Parapsychology Research Report for the National Research Council."

4. Y. Ikemi, S. Nakagawa, et al. (1975), "Psychosomatic Considerations on Cancer Patients Who Have Made a Narrow Escape from Death." *Dynamic Psychiatry* 31: 77–92.

5. A. Ulanov and B. Ulanov, *Primary Speech: A Psychology of Prayer* (Atlanta: John Knox Press, 1982).

6. L. Dossey, M.D., *Healing Words*.

10 Growing Beyond Your Fears

1. S. Jeffers, *Feel the Fear and Do It Anyway* (New York: Fawcett Books, 1992).

2. S. Ostrander, L. Schroeder, N. Ostrander, *Superlearning 2000* (New York: Delacorte Press, 1994).

11 Self-esteem: The Key to a Successful Pregnancy

1. R. H. Schuller, *Believe in the God Who Believes in You* (Nashville: Thomas Nelson Publishers, 1989).

2. N. Branden, *The Psychology of Self-esteem* (New York: Bantam Books, 1987).

3. S. Vannoy, *The 10 Greatest Gifts I Give My Children: Parenting from the Heart* (New York: Simon & Schuster, 1994).

4. A. Robbins, *Awaken the Giant Within: How to Take Immediate Control of Your Mental, Emotional, Physical, and Financial Destiny!* (New York: Simon & Schuster, 1992).

12 Setting the Goal to Live Responsibly

1. B. Tracy, *The Psychology of Achievement* (Niles, Il.: Nightingale-Conant Co., 1989).

14 Changing Behaviors

1. J. O. Prochaska, Ph.D., J. C. Norcross, Ph.D., C. C. Diclemente, Ph.D., *Changing for Good: The Revolutionary Program That Explains the Six Stages of Change and Teaches You How to Free Yourself from Bad Habits* (New York: William Morrow, 1994).

15 Good Communication Builds Strong Bonds: What You Can Do Now

1. Dennis Stott (1973), "Follow-up Study from Birth of the Effects of Prenatal Stresses." *Developmental Medicine and Child Neurology* 15: 770–87.

16 Nurturing Your Unborn Child Through Communication with Your Life Partner

1. V. Satir, *Conjoint Family Therapy* (Palo Alto, Calif.: Science and Behavior Books, 1967).
2. L. Gordon, Ph.D., *Love Knots: A Laundry List of Marital Mishaps, Marital Knots, Etc.* (New York: Dell, 1990).
3. George Bach and P. Wyden, *The Intimate Enemy* (New York: Avon Books, 1968).
4. George Bach and L. Torbet, *The Inner Enemy* (New York: William Morrow, 1983).

17 Learning to Fight Fairly

1. L. Gordon, Ph.D., *Passage to Intimacy: Key Concepts and Skills from the PAIRS Program Which Has Helped Thousands of Couples Rekindle Their Love* (New York: Simon & Schuster, 1993).
2. J. Gray, Ph.D., *Men Are from Mars, Women Are from Venus: A Practical Guide for Improving Communication and Getting What You Want in Your Relationships* (New York: HarperCollinsPublishers, 1992).
3. H. Hendrix, Ph.D., *Getting the Love You Want: A Guide for Couples* (New York: Harper & Row, 1988).

19 Creating Fetal Love Breaks by Putting It All Together

1. S. Covey, *The Seven Habits of Highly Effective People: Powerful Lessons in Personal Change* (New York: Fireside Publishers, 1989).
2. H. Benson, M.D., *The Relaxation Response* (New York: Avon, 1990).
3. Norman Vincent Peale, *Positive Imaging: The Powerful Way to Change Your Life* (New York: Ballantine, 1996).
4. Mark 11:24, New Revised Standard Version.

$\mathcal{I}$ndex